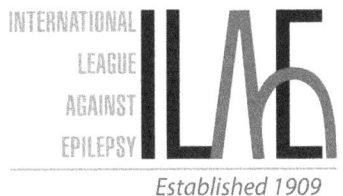
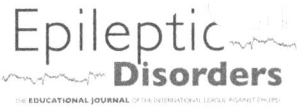

Established 1909

Epilepsy and cannabinoids

Alexis Arzimanoglou
Ulrich Brandl
Helen J. Cross
Antonio Gil-Nagel
Lieven Lagae
Cecilie Johannessen Landmark
Nicola Specchio
Elizabeth Thiele

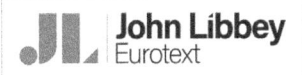

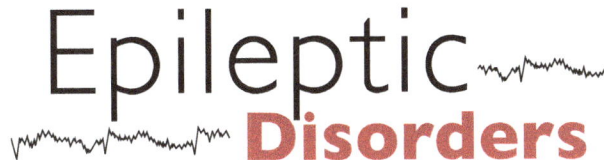

The Educational Journal of the International League Against Epilepsy
HTTP://WWW.EPILEPTICDISORDERS.COM

Editors-In-Chief

Alexis A. Arzimanoglou
Professor, Epilepsy Research Coordinator,
Hospital Sant Joan de Déu, Universitat de Barcelona, Spain
Head of Department of Paediatric Clinical Epileptology,
Sleep Disorders and Functional Neurology,
University Hospitals of Lyon, France
Sándor Beniczky
Professor, Aarhus University Hospital, Aarhus, Denmark
Head of Clinical Neurophysiology Department, Danish Epilepsy Centre, Dianalund, Denmark

Founding Editor

Jean Aicardi
Paris, France

Associate Editors

Ingmar Blümcke
Erlangen, Germany
Michael Duchowny
Miami, USA
Yushi Inoue
Shizuoka, Japan

Philippe Kahane
Grenoble, France
Rüdiger Köhling
Rostock, Germany
Michalis Koutroumanidis
London, UK

Doug Nordli
Los Angeles, USA
Lieven Lagae
Leuven, Belgium
Guido Rubboli
Dianalund, Denmark

Graeme Sills
Liverpool, UK
Mary-Lou Smith
Toronto, Canada
Pierre Thomas
Nice, France

Torbjörn Tomson
Stockholm, Sweden

Editorial Board

Nadia Bahi-Buisson
Paris, France
Carmen Barba
Florence, Italy
Fabrice Bartolomei
Marseille, France
Thomas Bast
Kork, Germany
Patricia Braga
Montevideo, Uruguay
Kees Braun
Utrecht, The Netherlands
Roberto Caraballo
Buenos Aires, Argentina
Mar Carreno
Barcelona, Spain

Francine Chassoux
Paris, France
Petia Dimova
Sofia, Bulgaria
David Dunn
Indianapolis, USA
Andras Fogarasi
Budapest, Hungary
Giuseppe Gobbi
Bologna, Italy
Jean Gotman
Montreal, Canada
Gregory Holmes
Vermont, USA
Hans Holthausen
Vogtareuth, Germany

Andres Kanner
Miami, USA
Katsuhiro Kobayashi
Okayama, Japan
Gaetan Lesca
Lyon, France
Shih-Hui Lim
Singapore
Andrew Lux
Bristol, UK
Stefano Meletti
Modena, Italy
Mohamad Mikati
Durham, USA
Fàbio A. Nascimento
Texas, USA

André Palmini
Porto Alegre, Brazil
Georgia Ramantani
Zürich, Switzerland
Aleksandar Ristic
Belgrade, Serbia
Ingrid Scheffer
Melbourne, Australia
Sanjay Sisodiya
London, UK
Mary Lou Smith
Toronto, Canada
Laura Tassi
Milan, Italy
Chong Tin Tan
Kuala Lumpur, Malaysia

Pierangelo Veggiotti
Pavia, Italy
Anna Maria Vezzani
Milan, Italy
Flavio Villani
Milan, Italy
Jo Wilmshurst
Cape Town, South Africa

ILAE Executive Committee

Samuel Wiebe, President
Calgary, Canada
Alla Guekht, Vice President
Moscow, Russian Federation
**Edward H. Bertram,
Secretary General**
Charlottesville, VA, USA
J. Helen Cross, Treasurer
London, UK
Emilio Perucca, Past President
Pavia, Italy

Angelina Kakooza
Kampala, Uganda
Akio Ikeda
Kyoto, Japan
Eugen Trinka
Salzburg, Austria
Chahnez Triki
Sfax, Tunisia
Roberto Caraballo
Buenos Aires, Argentina

Nathalie Jetté
New York, NY, USA
Astrid Nehlig
Paris, France
Michael Sperling
Philadelphia, PA, USA
Alexis Arzimanoglou
Lyon, France
Aristea Galanopoulou
New York, NY, USA

Shichuo Li
Beijing, China
Nicola Maggio
Tel Aviv, Israel
Xuefeng Wang
Chongqing, China
Jean Gotman
Montreal, Canada
**Martin Brodie,
IBE President**
Glasgow, Scotland

**Mary Secco,
IBE Secretary General**
London, Ontario, Canada
**Anthony Zimba,
IBE Treasurer**
Lusaka, Zambia

Editorial & Production Staff

MANAGING EDITOR
Oliver Gubbay
epileptic.disorders@gmail.com

PUBLICATIONS DIRECTOR
Gilles Cahn
gilles.cahn@jle.com

DESK EDITOR
Marine Rivière
marine.riviere@jle.com

PRODUCT MANAGER
Arnaud Cobo
arnaud.cobo@jle.com

ADVERTISING DIRECTOR
Noëlle Croisat
noelle.croisat@jle.com

ISBN : 978-2-7420-1633-4
ISSN : 1294-9361

Published by
Éditions John Libbey Eurotext
30 A rue Berthollet
Arcueil
www.jle.com

John Libbey Eurotext Plc
United Kingdom

© 2020, John Libbey Eurotext. All rights reserved.

Unauthorized duplication contravenes applicable laws.
It is prohibited to reproduce this work or any part of it without the authorization of the publisher or of the Centre Français d'Exploitation du Droit de Copie (CFC), 20, rue des Grands-Augustins, 75006 Paris.

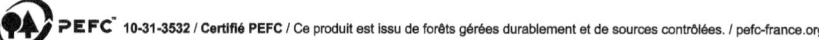 10-31-3532 / Certifié PEFC / Ce produit est issu de forêts gérées durablement et de sources contrôlées. / pefc-france.org

Contents

List of authors VII

The Cannabinoids International Experts Panel IX

Preface XI

Source of cannabinoids: what is available, what is used,
and where does it come from?
   Nicola Specchio, Nicola Pietrafusa, Helen J. Cross 1

The proposed mechanisms of action of CBD in epilepsy
   Royston A. Gray, Benjamin J. Whalley 11

Pharmacology and drug interactions of cannabinoids
   Cecilie Johannessen Landmark, Ulrich Brandl 17

The role of cannabinoids in epilepsy treatment:
a critical review of efficacy results from clinical trials
   Rima Nabbout, Elizabeth A. Thiele 25

Adverse effects of cannabinoids
   Carla Anciones, Antonio Gil-Nagel 33

Long-term effects of cannabinoids on development/behaviour
   Lieven Lagae 37

Epilepsy and cannabidiol: a guide to treatment
   Alexis Arzimanoglou, Ulrich Brandl, J. Helen Cross, Antonio Gil-Nagel,
   Lieven Lagae, Cecilie Johannessen Landmark, Nicola Specchio,
   Rima Nabbout, Elizabeth A. Thiele, Oliver Gubbay, on behalf
   ot The Cannabinoids International Experts Panel 43

Bibliography 59

List of authors

Carla Anciones, Epilepsy Program, Neurology Department, Hospital Ruber Internacional, Madrid, Spain

Alexis Arzimanoglou, Paediatric Clinical Epileptology, Sleep Disoorders and Functional Neurology Department, University Hospitals of Lyon, France and Hospital San Juan de Dios Children's Hospital, Barcelona, Spain, Members of the ERN EpiCARE

Ulrich Brandl, Department of Neuropediatrics, University Hospital Jena, Jena, Germany

Helen J. Cross, UCL-Institute of Child Health, Great Ormond Street Hospital for Children, Member of the European Reference Network EpiCARE, London & Young Epilepsy, Lingfield, UK

Antonio Gil-Nagel, Epilepsy Program, Neurology Department, Hospital Ruber Internacional, Madrid, Spain

Royston A. Gray, GW Research Ltd, Chivers Way, Histon, Cambridge, United Kingdom

Oliver Gubbay, Managing Editor, ILAE educational journal Epileptic Disorders, France

Cecilie Johannessen Landmark, Programme for Pharmacy, Faculty of Health Sciences, Oslo Metropolitan University, and The National center for epilepsy and Dpt of Pharmacology, Oslo University Hospital, Norway

Lieven Lagae, Paediatric Neurology, UZ Leuven, Member of the European Reference Network EpiCARE, Leuven, Belgium

Nicola Pietrafusa, Rare and Complex Epilepsy Unit, Department of Neurosciences, Bambino Gesù Children's Hospital, IRCCS, Member of the European Reference Network EpiCARE, Rome, Italy

Rima Nabbout, Department of Pediatric Neurology, Necker Enfants Malades Hospital, Reference Centre for Rare Epilepsies and Member of the ERN EpiCARE, Imagine Institute UMR1163, Paris Descartes University, Paris, France

Nicola Specchio, Rare and Complex Epilepsy Unit, Department of Neurosciences, Bambino Gesù Children's Hospital, IRCCS, Member of the European Reference Network EpiCARE, Rome, Italy

Elizabeth A. Thiele, Department of Neurology, Massachusetts General Hospital, Boston, USA

Benjamin J. Whalley, GW Research Ltd, Chivers Way, Histon, Cambridge, United Kingdom

The Cannabinoids International Experts Panel

Alexis Arzimanoglou (France), Stéphane Auvin (France), Ulrich Brandl (Germany), Mar Carreno (Spain), Richard Chin (UK), Roberta Cilio (Belgium), J. Helen Cross (UK), Vincenzo Di Marzo (Italy), Maria del Carmen Fons (Spain), Antonio Gil-Nagel (Spain), Elaine Hughes (USA), Floor Janssen (The Netherlands), Reetta Kalvilainen (Finland), Lieven Lagae (Belgium), Tally Lerman-Sagie (Israel), Maria Mazurkiewicz-Bełdzińska (Poland), Rima Nabbout (France), Nicola Pietrafusa (Italy), Georgia Ramantani (Switzerland), Sylvain Rheims (France), Rocio Sánchez-Carpintero (Spain), Nicola Specchio (Italy), Pasquale Striano (Italy), Elizabeth Thiele (USA)

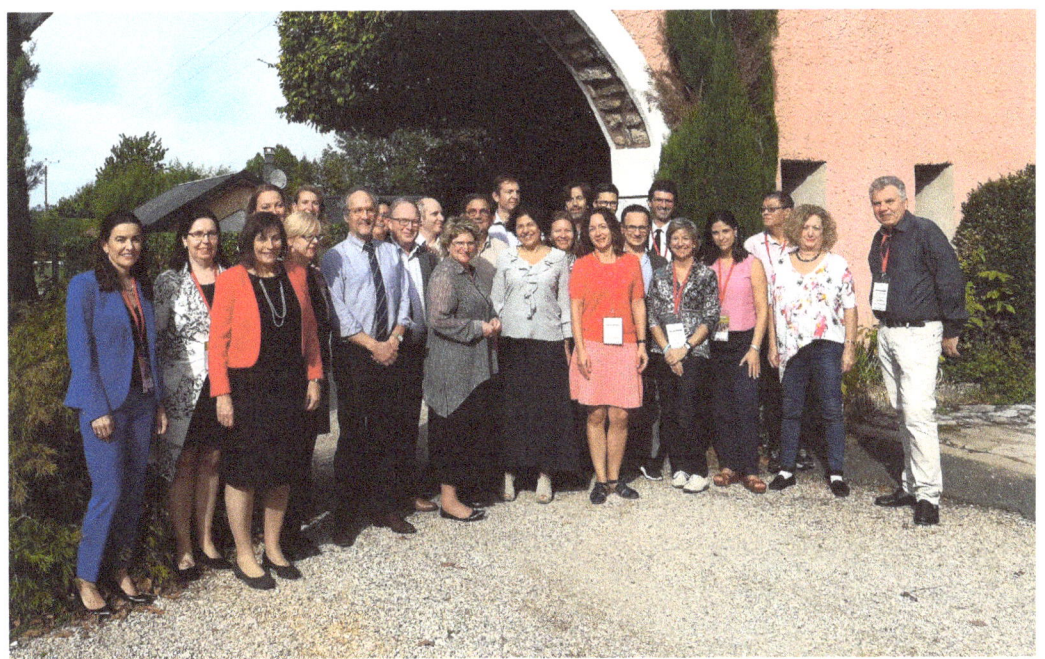

Preface

The growing interest in cannabidiol (CBD), specifically a pure form of CBD, as a treatment for epilepsy, among other conditions, is reflected in recent changes in legislation in some countries. Although there has been much speculation about the therapeutic value of cannabis based products as an anti-seizure treatment for some time, it is only within the last two years that Class I evidence has been available for a pure form of CBD, based on placebo-controlled RCTs for patients with Lennox-Gastaut syndrome and Dravet syndrome.

However, just as we are beginning to understand the significance of CBD as a treatment for epilepsy, in recent years, a broad spectrum of products advertised to contain CBD has emerged on the market. The effects of these products are fundamentally dependent on the purity, preparation, and concentration of CBD and other components, and consensus and standardisation are severely lacking regarding their preparation, composition, usage and effectiveness.

The availability of cannabis-based products and cannabinoid-based medicines, together with current regulations regarding indications in Europe (as of July 2019) is reviewed.

While the mechanism of action of CBD underlying the reduction of seizures in humans is unknown, CBD possesses affinity for multiple targets, across a range of target classes, resulting in functional modulation of neuronal excitability, relevant to the pathophysiology of many disease types, including epilepsy. The pharmacological data supporting the role of three such targets, namely Transient receptor potential vanilloid-1 (TRPV1), the orphan G protein-coupled receptor-55 (GPR55) and the equilibrative nucleoside transporter 1 (ENT-1) are discussed.

Cannabinoids include a variety of substances, of which CBD is the main substance investigated for the treatment of epilepsy. CBD preparations exist in various forms. There are significant differences in quality control regarding content and reproducibility for an approved drug versus herbal preparations. Cannabidiol has challenging pharmacological properties, and pharmaceutical and pharmacokinetic aspects will depend on the formulation or preparation of a certain product. The characteristics, pharmacokinetic challenges, and interactions of standardised CBD-containing drugs based on evidence from clinical and pharmacokinetic studies are presented. We detail the clinical studies using purified CBD (Epidiolex/Epidyolex), including the first open interventional exploratory study and Randomized Control Ttrials for Dravet and Lennox-Gastaut syndromes. Results of these trials led to the FDA and EMA approval, respectively in 2018 and 2019, for the treatment of seizures associated with these two rare epilepsy syndromes in patients two years of age and older.

Cannabidiol is a generally well tolerated drug with transitory, dose-dependent mild to moderate effects like somnolence, decreased appetite or diarrhoea. However, severe life-threatening reactions can also rarely occur, and are often related to the noncontrolled toxic combination with other antiseizure drugs that are widely used in this type of patients like sodium valproate or clobazam. Adverse effects observedin clinical trials are presented and their management in clinical prractice discussed.

Long-term studies, using large childhood epilepsy cohorts, of cannabinoids on neurodevelopment and behaviour are still needed. The indirect evidence obtained from the randomised controlled trials with cannabidiol, data on the consequences of prenatal cannabis exposure, and data on the effect of adolescent cannabis use are presented. No hard conclusions can be drawn, mainly because of methodological problems (dosage of THC and other cannabis-derived products, duration of exposure, concordant addiction to other drugs, genetic factors, educational level, etc.), however, long-term data show a possible negative and lasting effect on cognitive and especially behavioural functions. Externalising behavioural problems and a decrease in IQ have been reported as a result of chronic cannabis use.

In contrast, purified CBD, is a standardised pharmaceutical preparation that is subject to minimal variability. Given the range of different seizure types associated with Dravet Syndrome, Lennox-Gastaut syndrome or epilepsy as an expression of the Tuberous Sclerosis Complex, CBD would appear to have a favourable effect on a large spectrum of seizures namely clonic, myoclonic, myoclonic-astatic, and generalised tonic-clonic seizures.

Based on an International Experts Workshop on Cannabinoids in Epilepsy, held in France, the aim of this book is to provide information to adult and child neurologists and epileptologists on the therapeutic value of CBD products, principally a purified form, in routine practice for patients with drug-resistant epilepsy.

Source of cannabinoids: what is available, what is used and where does it come from?

Nicola Specchio, Nicola Pietrafusa, Helen J. Cross

Currently, cannabis-based medications are widely perceived to represent an alternative therapeutic strategy for many different diseases, approved from 2011 in many European countries (Abuhasira *et al.*, 2018). That aside, they do not represent a single compound. The Cannabis plant contains about 565 compounds, among which 120 are cannabinoids (ElSohly *et al.*, 2017). The most abundant of these are cannabidiol (CBD) and delta-9-tetrahydrocannabinol (THC). THC, a partial agonist of cannabinoid type 1 (CB1) receptors, mostly located in the brain in the inhibitory (GABA)ergic and excitatory glutamatergic neurons, is responsible for the psychoactive effects (Hill *et al.*, 2012).

Cannabinoids are used in many fields of medicine (*table 1*: some examples are spasticity (*e.g.* multiple sclerosis) (Lynch and Campbell, 2011), chronic pain (*e.g.* oncologic and neuropathic pain) (Noyes *et al.*, 1975; Bestard and Toth, 2011; Aggarwal and Blinderman, 2014) resistant to corticosteroids or opioids (Aggarwal and Blinderman, 2014), chemotherapy-related nausea and vomiting (Smith *et al.*, 2015), cachexia and anorexia in patients with cancer or AIDS (Beal *et al.*, 1997), glaucoma resistant to conventional therapies (Tomida *et al.*, 2006), facial and body movements associated with Gilles de la Tourette syndrome (Müller-Vahl, 2013), and many other clinical conditions (Holdcroft *et al.*, 1997, 2006; Tomida *et al.*, 2006; Skrabek *et al.*, 2008; Robbins *et al.*, 2009). Sativex (oromucosal spray THC/CBD 1:1) is a therapeutic add-on option, approved for un-responsive spasticity in multiple sclerosis patients, used in several European countries (Barnes, 2006). Several studies suggest that CBD can be also effective for neuropsychiatric disorders, including anxiety and schizophrenia (Russo, 2008; Rong *et al.*, 2017). CBD may also be effective in treating post-traumatic stress disorder and may have anxiolytic, antipsychotic, antiemetic, and anti-inflammatory properties (Borgelt *et al.*, 2013; Whiting *et al.*, 2015; Pisanti *et al.*, 2017).

Table 1. Applications of CBD.

- Epilepsy
- Neuropsychiatric disorders:
  – anxiety
  – schizophrenia
  – post-traumatic stress disorders
  – anxiolytic
  – antipsychotic
- Antiemetic
- Anti-inflammatory properties

Cannabis use has become increasingly prevalent in patients with epilepsy. In animal models, THC has primarily anticonvulsant properties but is pro-convulsant in some species (Devinsky et al., 2014). The molecule most studied for the treatment of epilepsy is CBD (Friedman and Devinsky, 2016). Anecdotal reports of individual children with drug-resistant epilepsy who appeared to have a miraculous response to CBD-enriched oils has fuelled public interest. In 2013, a five-year-old girl named Charlotte, with *SCN1A*-confirmed Dravet syndrome (DS) and up to 50 generalized tonic-clonic seizures daily, obtained a greater than 90% reduction in her seizures after three months of treatment with high-CBD-strain cannabis extract (later marketed as "Charlotte's Web") (Maa and Figi, 2014).

Subsequently, Porter and Jacobson reported on an internet-based survey in which 84% of parents who had administered CBD-enriched cannabis extract to 19 children with intractable epilepsy reported a significant reduction in seizure frequency (Porter and Jacobson, 2013). In 2015, Hussain et al. (2015) conducted a survey with similar results. Similar case reports, surveys, and small retrospective chart reviews suggested CBD may improve seizure control, alertness, mood, and sleep (Schonhofen et al., 2018).

This phenomenon has encouraged a high level of interest among physicians, medicinal chemists, pharmaceutical companies, and the general population, and led to impassioned pleas from families with children with severe epilepsy for access to cannabis derivatives (Filloux, 2015).

In January 2016, a retrospective Israeli study describing the effect of CBD-enriched medical cannabis on children with epilepsy was published (Tzadok et al., 2016). In this study, 74 patients with intractable epilepsy were enrolled and started on cannabis oil extract, continued for at least three months (average: six months). The selected formula contained CBD and THC at a ratio of 20:1 in olive oil. Seizure frequency was assessed according to a parental report during clinic visits. The results showed a reduction in seizure frequency in 89% of all children enrolled, with improvement in behaviour and alertness, language, communication, motor skills, and sleep.

In a recent meta-analysis (Pamplona et al., 2018), the data from 11 studies provided strong evidence in support of the therapeutic value of high-CBD treatments (CBD-rich cannabis extracts/purified CBD), at least as far as this population of 670 patients was concerned; patients treated with CBD-rich extracts reported a lower average dose (6.1 mg/kg/day) than those using purified CBD (27.1 mg/kg/day).

Randomised controlled trials of pharmaceutically prepared CBD have shown benefit for DS and Lennox Gastaut syndrome (LGS) (Devinsky et al., 2017, 2018; Thiele et al., 2018, 2019). Studies are underway to evaluate CBD efficacy for a broader range of epilepsy syndromes and more than 20 trials are currently listed on ClinicalTrials.gov.

■ Products available

The US Food and Drug Administration (FDA) has approved Epidiolex (GW Pharma) CBD oral solution for the treatment of seizures associated with LGS and DS, in patients two years of age and older (FDA, 2018) In July 2019, the European Medicines Agency (EMA) granted marketing authorisation for Epidyolex, "indicated for use as adjunctive therapy of seizures associated with LGS or DS, in conjunction with clobazam, for patients two years of age and older". Detailed recommendations will be published following marketing authorisation by the European Commission (European Medicines Agency, 2019).

In anticipation of the commercialization of Epidyolex in Europe, the spectrum of medical cannabis products for epilepsy is significantly large. Artisanal cannabis products with variable ratios of CBD:THC soon became available across many countries and states. Users obtained products from government dispensaries and through internet purchasing (including Charlotte's Web). Public interest in CBD products has partly been based on the belief that "natural" products may be safer with fewer adverse effects than conventional AEDs.

To date, several galenic products are available, according to European Pharmacopeia: cannabis decoction filter bags, unit dose formulation for inhalation, and cannabis extracts, mainly in olive oil.

Cannabis based preparations are mainly distinguished as CBD dietary supplements, and "CBD-enriched oils", obtained from extraction of different *Cannabis sativa L.* chemotypes with high content of CBD, are the most popular products used. CBD is not a controlled substance in the European Union; several companies produce and distribute CBD-based products obtained from inflorescences of industrial hemp varieties. No analytical controls are mandatory and no legal protection or guarantees about the composition and quality, nor obligatory testing or basic regulatory framework to determine indication area, daily dosage, route of administration, maximum recommended daily dose, packaging, shelf life, and stability are required.

Magistral preparations from cannabis plants are more acceptable and have been approved by 10 more European countries (Abuhasira *et al.*, 2018). Most of the regulators allow physicians to decide on the specific indications for prescription of cannabis-based products, but some regulators dictate only few specific indications. As opposed to herbal cannabis, cannabinoid-based medicines are authorized by the FDA and by most of the countries in Europe. Many countries have changed their legislation about medical cannabis in recent years and it is likely that the regulations will continue to change in the future. It should be noted that in many countries, there is a considerable gap between official authorization, which may be quite permissive, to actual access of patients to medical cannabis (Abuhasira *et al.*, 2018).

Galenical "CBD oil" is prepared by pharmacists following medical prescriptions in several European Union countries such as Germany, Italy and Holland. The German Drug Codex (DAC), which is published by the Federal Union of German Associations of Pharmacists (ABDA) and functions as a supplementary book to the Pharmacopoeia, suggests a preparation of 5 % CBD in medium chain triglyceride oil, also indicating detailed analytical controls of galenic preparations (DAC, 2015). Six different varieties are available on the market in Europe, with standardized THC and CBD concentrations: Bedrocan, Bedrobinol, Bediol (from *C. sativa*, with 22%; 13.5% and 6.5% mean THC and <1%, <1% and 8% mean CBD, respectively), Bedica (from *C. indica*, with 14% THC and <1% CBD), Bedrolite (from *C. sativa*, with approximately 0.4% THC and 9% CBD) and Bedropuur (from *C. indica*, with high-THC and <1% CBD).

Poor levels of standardization are currently applied to the galenic preparation of cannabis oil extracts and there is a lack of regulatory measures that have resulted in insufficient quality control of artisanal preparations. Laboratory analyses have shown that most products have significantly different contents of individual cannabinoids compared with their marketing label (Vandrey *et al.*, 2015). Carcieri *et al.* (2018) highlighted broad variability in THC and CBD concentrations, and showed that the interlot variability in extraction yields was higher for Bedrocan-based preparations, whereas Bediol-based preparations showed significantly higher extraction yields for both THC (compared to Bedrocan) and CBD (compared to Bedrolite).

Analytical controls are not mandatory for CBD-based products, leaving consumers with no legal protection or guarantees about the composition and quality of the product they are acquiring. Currently, CBD-based products are not subject to any obligatory testing or basic regulatory framework to determine the indication area, daily dosage, route of administration, maximum recommended daily dose, packaging, shelf life, or stability (*box 1*).

Among the above-mentioned strains, Bedrolite with CBD and THC contents of 9% and <1%, respectively, is frequently used for the preparation of galenic "CBD-based oil". Moreover, pharmacies are allowed to distribute CBD oils obtained from hemp but declared as additives or aromatic preparations if produced in Italy, or designed as dietary supplement if imported from other European countries. "CBD-enriched oils", obtained from extraction of different *Cannabis sativa* L. chemotypes with high content of CBD, are the most popular products used.

Since CBD, in contrast to THC, is not a controlled substance in the European Union, several companies produce and distribute CBD-based products obtained from inflorescences of industrial hemp varieties. The extraction procedure is called "supercritical CO_2 extraction", which provides an extract rich in CBD from the cannabis. There are different biological active compounds that can be isolated during the extract procedures: omega-3 fatty acids, vitamins, terpenes, flavonoids, and other phytocannabinoids such as cannabichromene (CBC), cannabigerol (CBG), cannabinol (CBN), and cannabidivarian (CBCV) (Calvi *et al.*, 2018). During the extraction procedure, non-cannabinoid compounds are also isolated. Terpenes represent the largest group (more than 100 different molecules) of cannabis phytochemicals. These compounds have the ability to easily cross cell membranes and the blood-brain barrier. An entourage effect between cannabinoids and terpenes as a result of synergistic action has been hypothesized (Russo, 2011; Aizpurua-Olaizola *et al.*, 2016).

With regards to cannabis macerated oils, there are major concerns about correct preparation methods and conditions regarding the evolution of major and minor compounds (can-

---

Box 1. CBD is not a controlled substance in the European Union

Several companies produce and distribute CBD-based products obtained from inflorescences of industrial hemp varieties.
- No analytical controls are mandatory;
- No legal protection or guarantees about the composition and quality;
- No obligatory testing or basic regulatory framework to determine:
  - indication area;
  - daily dosage;
  - route of administration;
  - maximum recommended daily dose;
  - packaging;
  - shelf life;
  - stability.

nabis and terpenes) during storage in order to define the ideal shelf-life (including storage temperature). Pavlovic et al. (2018) demonstrated, by analysing CBD oils commercially available in European countries, a high degree of variability of CBD concentrations in commercialized CBD oil preparations. The quality of 14 CBD oil preparations produced in different European countries and purchased on the internet was evaluated. Bedrolite macerated oil prepared as a galenic product was used as a reference therapeutic formulation. Nine out of the 14 samples studied had concentrations that differed notably from the declared amount, while CBD for the remaining five was within optimal limits (variation <10%).

Overall, we might conclude that there is a huge variation in the quality and safety of the CBD-based preparations available on the market. Clear labelling regarding the exact concentration of CBD is not yet mandatory, CBD concentrations are not always in accordance with producer information, and there is extreme variability in the commercialized CBD oil preparations, justifying the need for stricter regulations/controls.

One further study has been published with similar results (Bonn-Miller et al., 2017). The aim of this article was to advise how to read CBD/cannabinoid product labels. Through an internet search with the following keywords, "CBD", "cannabidiol", "oil", "tincture", and "vape", performed between September 12, 2016, and October 15, 2016, CBD products available for online retail purchase that included CBD content on the packaging were identified. Eighty-four products were purchased and analysed. Observed CBD concentration ranged between 0.10 mg/mL and 655.27 mg/mL (median: 9.45 mg/mL). Median labelled concentration was 15.00 mg/mL (range: 1.33-800.00 mg/mL). With respect to CBD, 42.85% (95% CI : 32.82%-53.53%) of products were under-labelled (n = 36), 26.19% (95% CI : 17.98%-36.48%) were over-labelled (n = 22), and 30.95% (95% CI: 22.08%-41.49%) were accurately labelled (n = 26). The 26% of products that contained less CBD than labelled could have negated any potential clinical response. The level of CBD in the over-labelled products in this study is similar in magnitude to levels that triggered warning letters to 14 businesses in 2015-2016 from the US Food and Drug Administration (i.e. actual CBD content was negligible or less than 1% of the labelled content), suggesting that there is a continued need for federal and state regulatory agencies to take steps to ensure accuracy of labelling of these consumer products. Under-labelling is less concerning as CBD appears to neither have abuse liability nor serious adverse consequences at high doses, however, the THC content observed may be sufficient to produce intoxication or impairment, especially among children. Although the exclusive procurement of products online is a study limitation given the frequently changing online marketplace, these products represent the most readily available to US consumers. Additional monitoring should be conducted to determine changes in this marketplace over time and to compare internet products with those sold in dispensaries. These findings highlight the need for manufacturing and testing standards, as well as oversight of medicinal cannabis products.

We performed a survey in Italy with questions outlined in *table 2*. In Italy, all the above-mentioned products are available, together with some further products: *i.e.* HEMPY® CBD OIL 5%-10%-50% ; FM2 (Military Pharmaceutical Institute of Florence), 5-8% THC and 7-12% CBD from C. *Sativa* ; and FM1 (Military Pharmaceutical Institute of Florence), 13-20% THC and <1% CBD from C. *Sativa*. The most frequent products

Table 2. Questions included in a survey related to the available CBD products in Italy.

What forms of therapeutic cannabis are available in your country ?
Bedrocan (19% THC and < 1% CBD, from *C. Sativa*)
Bedrobinol (12% THC and <1% CBD, from *C. Sativa*)
Bediol (6% THC and 7.5% CBD, from *C. Sativa*)
Bedrolite (<0.4% THC and 9% CBD, from *C. Sativa*)
Bedica (14% THC and <1% CBD, from *C. Indica*)
Pedanios 22/1 (22% THC and <1% CBD, from *C. Sativa*)
Pedanios 8 (8% THC and 8% CBD, from *C. Indica*)
Pedanios 1/8 (<1% THC and 8% CBD, from *C. Ibrida*)
Crystals 99% pure CBD
Others (specify)
What is used in your centre for epilepsy ?
Which formulation do you use in your centre ?
What dose do you use ?
Where does it come from ?
Are hemp oils a concern ?
What is the relative evidence for dose/safety ?

used are Bedrolite, Pedanios 1/8, and above all CBD crystals 99%. All are very slowly titrated, and CBD crystals 99% are used at a dose of 2-25 mg/kg/day. Bedrolite originates from Holland, Pedanios from Canada, and FM1/2 from Italy. There is no evidence related to guidance on dose and relative safety. Regarding reimbursement, therapeutic cannabis costs around 9 euros per gram, and CBD crystal 99% oil costs around 20-25 euros for 10 mL at 5%. Cannabis can be prescribed free of charge for any pathology that exists with accredited scientific documentation (according to the "Di Bella" law 94/98). The indications for free cannabinoids are multiple sclerosis, anorexia, vomiting and nausea from chemotherapy or HIV, glaucoma, Tourette's syndrome, and chronic pain. Only few regions in Italy is there also an indication for epilepsy. Any other indication outside these listed is subject to payment.

A recent US survey reported 19 parents using an artisanal preparation of CBD-enriched oil to treat their children with treatment-resistant epilepsy, aged between 12 and 16 years (Porter and Jacobson, 2013). Twelve of 19 had DS, four Doose syndrome, and one each with epilepsy in females with intellectual disability, LGS, and idiopathic epilepsy. Overall, the results showed that two patients were reported to be seizure-free (one with DS and one with Doose syndrome), eight patients had >80% reduction in seizure frequency (5/12 patients with DS), three had >50% reduction (all DS), three had >25% reduction, and three patients experienced no change (two DS and one with Doose syndrome). Up to 80% reported positive side effects (better mood, increased alertness, and better sleep). Less than a third reported negative side effects (drowsiness, fatigue, and reduced appetite), and severe side effects were not reported. Similar results were reported in a different study based on parental reporting of response to oral cannabis extracts in 2015 (Press *et al.*, 2015). Seventy-five patients were enrolled: 23% with DS and 89% with LGS. Fifty-seven percent reported no improvement in seizure control, and 33% reported a 50% reduction in seizures. If families had moved to Colorado for cannabis treatment, the responder rate was 47% but only 22% for those already living in Colorado. Adverse events occurred in 44% of the patients (increased seizures in 13% and somnolence and fatigue in 12%).

Legislation in different countries

The WHO Expert Committee on Drug Dependence recommended, on 24th January 2019, to the United Nations that preparations considered to be pure CBD should not be scheduled within the International Drug Control Conventions. The Committee proposed adding a footnote to the entry for "cannabis and cannabis resin" in Schedule 1 of the Single Convention on Narcotics Drugs of 1961 to specify that CBD preparations are not under international control. This recommendation was due to be considered by the UN Commission on Narcotic Drugs in March 2019, but the vote was postponed to allow member states more time to discuss the consequences of potential changes in scheduling of cannabis for national and international control measures[1].

The United Kingdom

A statement was issued by the Medicines and Healthcare products Regulatory Agency (MHRA) in 2016 that products containing CBD used for medical purposes are considered as a medicine, subject to standard licensing requirements (Medicines and Healthcare products Regulatory Agency, 2018). CBD with minimal THC (including Epidiolex®) is not a scheduled drug; cannabis-derived medicinal products containing >0.2% THC were, however, Schedule 1 and therefore required a Home Office licence to be utilised.

The Advisory Council on the Misuse of Drugs (ACMD) thereafter recommended that "cannabis-derived medicinal products of the appropriate standard" be moved out of Schedule 1 and, subject to further refinement of the definition of cannabis-based products for medicinal use, into Schedule 2. Synthetic cannabinoids were specifically excluded from this and reserved for further consideration. Moving cannabis-based products for medicinal use to Schedule 2 will mean those cannabis-based products can be prescribed medicinally where there is an unmet clinical need.

In light of the above, the UK Government has decided to lay regulations which will move cannabis-based products for medicinal use out of Schedule 1 and into Schedule 2 of the MDR, with the exception of synthetic cannabinoids. Subject to annulment by either House of Parliament, those regulations came into force on 1st November 2018. The Government has defined a cannabis-based product for medicinal use in humans as "a preparation or other product, other than one to which paragraph 5 of part 1 of Schedule 4 applies, which:

– is or contains cannabis, cannabis resin, cannabinol or a cannabinol derivative (not being dronabinol or its stereoisomers);
– is produced for medicinal use in humans;

---

[1] https://www.who.int/medicines/access/controlled-substances/WHOCBDReportMay2018-2.pdf

– and is (i) a medicinal product, or (ii) a substance or preparation for use as an ingredient of, or in the production of an ingredient of, a medicinal product".

Under the proposed new regime, all cannabis-based products for medicinal use apart from Sativex® (listed in Schedule 4 of the MDR and which has a market authorisation) would be unlicensed medicines[2].

United States of America

CBD is one of many cannabinoids present in cannabis, and as such is in Schedule 1 of the Controlled Substances Act (Schedule 1 is the most restricted/regulated drug class, reserved for medications with a high potential for abuse and no currently accepted medical use). The US FDA approved Epidiolex, the first ever drug derived from CBD, on June 25, 2018. Once approved by the FDA, the Drug Enforcement Administration (DEA) had 90 days to act since CBD is a Schedule 1 substance. On September 27, 2018, the DEA rescheduled Epidiolex as a Schedule 5 substance, which is in line with the FDA's recommendation. Schedule 5 drugs, substances, or chemicals are defined as drugs with lower potential for abuse[3].

Canada

CBD is specifically listed in "Cannabis, its preparations and derivatives" as a controlled substance, according to the Schedule 2 Controlled Drugs and Substances Act. However, in 2016, Canada's Access to Cannabis for Medical Purposes Regulations came into effect. These regulations improve access to cannabis used for medicinal purposes, including CBD (Government of Canada Justice Laws Website, 2017).

Australia

In 2015, CBD in preparations for therapeutic use, containing 2% or less of other cannabinoids found in cannabis, was placed in Schedule 4 as a "Prescription Only Medicine or Prescription Animal Remedy". Previous to this, it was placed in Schedule 9 as a prohibited substance (Australian Government Department of Health Therapeutic Goods Administration, 2017).

New Zealand

CBD is a controlled drug, however, by passing the Misuse of Drugs Amendment Regulations 2017 in September 2017, many of the restrictions currently imposed by the regulations have been removed since then. The changes will mean that CBD products, in which the level of other naturally occurring cannabinoids is less than 2% of the cannabinoid content, will be easier to access for medical use (New Zealand Government Ministry of Health, 2017).

---

[2] https://www.england.nhs.uk/wp-content/uploads/2018/10/letter-guidance-on-cannabis-based-products-for-medicinal-use.pdf
[3] https://www.fda.gov/news-events/press-announcements/fda-approves-first-drug-comprised-active-ingredient-derived-marijuana-treat-rare-severe-forms

Switzerland

CBD is not subject to the Narcotics Act because it does not produce a psychoactive effect. It is still subject to standard Swiss legislation (Swiss Agency for Therapeutic Products, 2017).

France

As of 8th June 2013, cannabis derivatives can be used in France for the manufacture of medicinal products. The products can only be obtained with a prescription and will only be prescribed when all other medications have failed to effectively relieve suffering. Hemp CBD oil containing less than (and up to) 0.2% THC is allowed. The Minister for Health announced in November 2017 that the presence of CBD in products for public consumption was authorised providing there is a maximum of 0.2% THC (French National Agency for Medicines and Health Products Safety, 2018).

Italy

The Ministry of Health (MoH), from November 2015, can issue licences for cultivation, production, possession, and use, and herbal cannabis may be prescribed with medical prescription. The use of cannabis is licenced only for symptomatic treatment, in cases in which traditional treatments have failed. Eligible conditions are primarily spasticity, chronic pain, nausea from chemotherapy or HIV treatments, loss of appetite from cancer or AIDS, glaucoma, and Gilles de la Tourette syndrome. Licensed farmers deliver the cannabis to the MoH, who then allocate it for production. The pharmacists buy the active substance from the MoH using vouchers, and prepare magistral preparations accordingly (EMCDDA, 2018). Physicians should prescribe appropriate products based on genetic strain, dispensing amount, and consumption method for each patient. Currently, all legal cannabis sold in Italian pharmacies is derived from Holland (import fixed at 750 Kg for 2019), Italian cultivation by the Military Chemical and Pharmaceutical Institute of Florence (estimated production of 200 kg), and Canada (import fixed at 100 kg for 2018) (Zaami *et al.*, 2018).

Conclusion

In conclusion, there is pronounced variability in CBD concentrations in commercialized CBD oil preparations. Differences in the overall cannabinoid profiles along with discrepancies in the terpene fingerprint justify the necessity to provide firmer regulation and control. Precise information regarding CBD oil composition is crucial for consumers, as individual doses throughout the administration period have to be adapted according to CBD bioavailability. This is of fundamental importance regarding consumer safety, as CBD oil preparations are used therapeutically, regardless of the fact that they are registered as dietary supplements.

The proposed mechanisms of action of CBD in epilepsy

Royston A. Gray, Benjamin J. Whalley

Cannabidiol (CBD) possesses affinity and functional agonist or antagonist activity at multiple 7-transmembrane receptors, ion channels, and neurotransmitter transporters (Ibeas et al. 2015). While a diverse pharmacology would be predicted, target engagement and subsequent therapeutic effect is dependent upon relevant systemic exposure to CBD. Thus, several targets are considered implausible based upon the low affinity and/or potency exhibited by CBD when compared to systemic exposures measured in the plasma of patients receiving therapeutic doses of purified CBD.

CBD has been shown to demonstrate positive effects against a wide spectrum of seizures based on animal model data (Klein et al., 2017). Of those targets where engagement is plausible, several have been investigated based upon their physiological relevance to maintaining normal neuronal function (e.g. membrane potential, neurotransmitter release and uptake, and postsynaptic calcium mobilization). While the precise mechanism of action of CBD in the control of epileptic seizures in humans remains unknown, recent evidence has focussed attention upon the following effects of CBD: modulation of intracellular Ca^{2+} (including effects on neuronal Ca^{2+} mobilization via GPR55 and influx via TRPV1) and modulation of adenosine-mediated signaling (*figure 1*). Here, we describe the pharmacological data supporting the roles of GPR55, TRPV1, and adenosine transport in the mechanism of action of CBD in the treatment of seizures in humans, as demonstrated by the ameliorations observed with CBD (Epidiolex in the US and Epidyolex in the EU) in Dravet and Lennox Gastaut syndromes (Devinsky et al., 2017, 2018; Thiele et al., 2018).

GPR55 was first identified as an orphan Class A G protein-coupled receptor (GPCR) enriched in brain (Sawzdargo et al., 1999) and was originally suggested as a novel cannabinoid receptor (Ryberg et al., 2007) and the subject of patent claims (Brown and Wise, 2001). However, poor sequence homology of GPR55 relative to CB_1 and CB_2 receptors, divergent pharmacology, and signal transduction suggest an alternative classification is appropriate, although at the time of writing, GPR55 remains an orphan receptor. GPR55 has been shown to utilize G_q, G_{12}, or G_{13} for signal transduction and the subsequent increased intracellular Ca^{2+} concentration through release of inositol triphosphate (IP3)-gated intracellular Ca^{2+} stores and activation of RhoA and phospholipase C.

In 2007, Ryberg et al. (2007) identified endogenous 2-arachidonylglycerol (2-AG), virodhamine (O-arachidonoyl ethanolamine), noladin ether (2-arachidonoyl glyceryl ether), oleoylethanolamide and palmitoylethanolamide (PEA), exogenous Δ^9-tetrahydrocannabinol (Δ^9-THC), and CP55940 as GPR55 agonists and first described CBD's antagonism of the GPR55 receptor. While the putative endogenous GPR55 receptor agonist, l-α-lysophosphatidylinositol (LPI), has been consistently described as a micromolar potency agonist of GPR55 (Kapur et al., 2009), up to, and since this finding, the pharmacology of

GPR55 has been the subject of significant investigation and has revealed emerging complexity.

As described by Sharir & Abood (2010), the molecular pharmacology of CBD at GPR55 is dependent upon the recombinant or endogenously expressing system and on the signalling system examined. The example pertinent to the present review is the observation that while CBD can antagonize LPI-induced, GPR55-mediated stimulation of GTPγS binding and ERK phosphorylation, no such effect on LPI-induced β-arrestin recruitment is observed. These data are suggestive of biased antagonism where the ligand, in this case CBD, possesses functional selectivity for G-protein-mediated cellular events over another. In the absence of convincing pharmacological data describing competition of LPI and CBD for the same binding site at the GPR55 receptor, this remains plausible. Furthermore, in native systems where LPI interacts with multiple molecular targets, it is possible that the apparent antagonism of LPI-mediated physiological effects by CBD may be through interaction with one or more of such targets, including GPR55.

Moreover, coupling the role of GPR55 in modulation of neuronal excitability to its involvement in the pathophysiology of seizure was bolstered by the observation that GPR55 receptor expression is increased in the epileptic hippocampus (Rosenberg et al., 2018).

Functional antagonism of GPR55 by purified CBD was investigated by examination of LPI-stimulated ERK1/2 phosphorylation in human GPR55-expressing HEK 293 cells. Purified CBD (1 μM) produced a parallel, rightward and marginally downward shift in the LPI concentration response curve, indicating functional antagonism of the GPR55 receptor. The primary evidence for the role of GPR55 in CBD's mechanism of action comes from studies in which the effect of LPI on neuronal excitability was assessed in acute hippocampal slice preparations. Here, the effect of purified CBD on LPI-induced GPR55-mediated modulation of mEPSC was assessed by whole-cell patch clamp recording in hippocampal slices from epileptic rats, sacrificed two weeks following a 60-minute episode of sustained pilocarpine-induced temporal lobe seizure and littermate, vehicle-treated controls. Activation of GPR55 by LPI increased mEPSC frequency in hippocampal slices, the magnitude of which was significantly greater in epileptic than non-epileptic rats. Since LPI effects on mEPSC frequency are transient, CBD was applied 20 minutes before LPI and functionally antagonized GPR55-mediated increases in mEPSC frequency in both non-epileptic and epileptic conditions.

Adenosine has been described as the endogenous modulator of neuronal excitability (Dunwiddie, 1980); and the brain's endogenous anticonvulsant and neuroprotectant (Weltha et al., 2018). The endogenous nucleoside adenosine is released locally upon cellular insult and mediates its physiological effects via interaction with four 7-transmenbrane G-protein-coupled receptors whose classification (A_1, A_{2a}, A_{2b}, and A_3) is based upon sequence homology and pharmacology. Each adenosine receptor subtype possesses a well-defined tissue distribution and second messenger coupling, reflecting their role in the modulation of neuronal excitability, inflammation, and cardiovascular function.

Given their expression in the CNS, in consideration of the role of adenosine as a negative modulator of excitatory transmission and therefore seizure termination, the key receptor subtypes of interest are A_1, A_{2a}, and A_3. The anticonvulsive effects of adenosine are largely attributable to the activation of pre- and postsynaptic Gi/o protein-coupled adenosine A_1

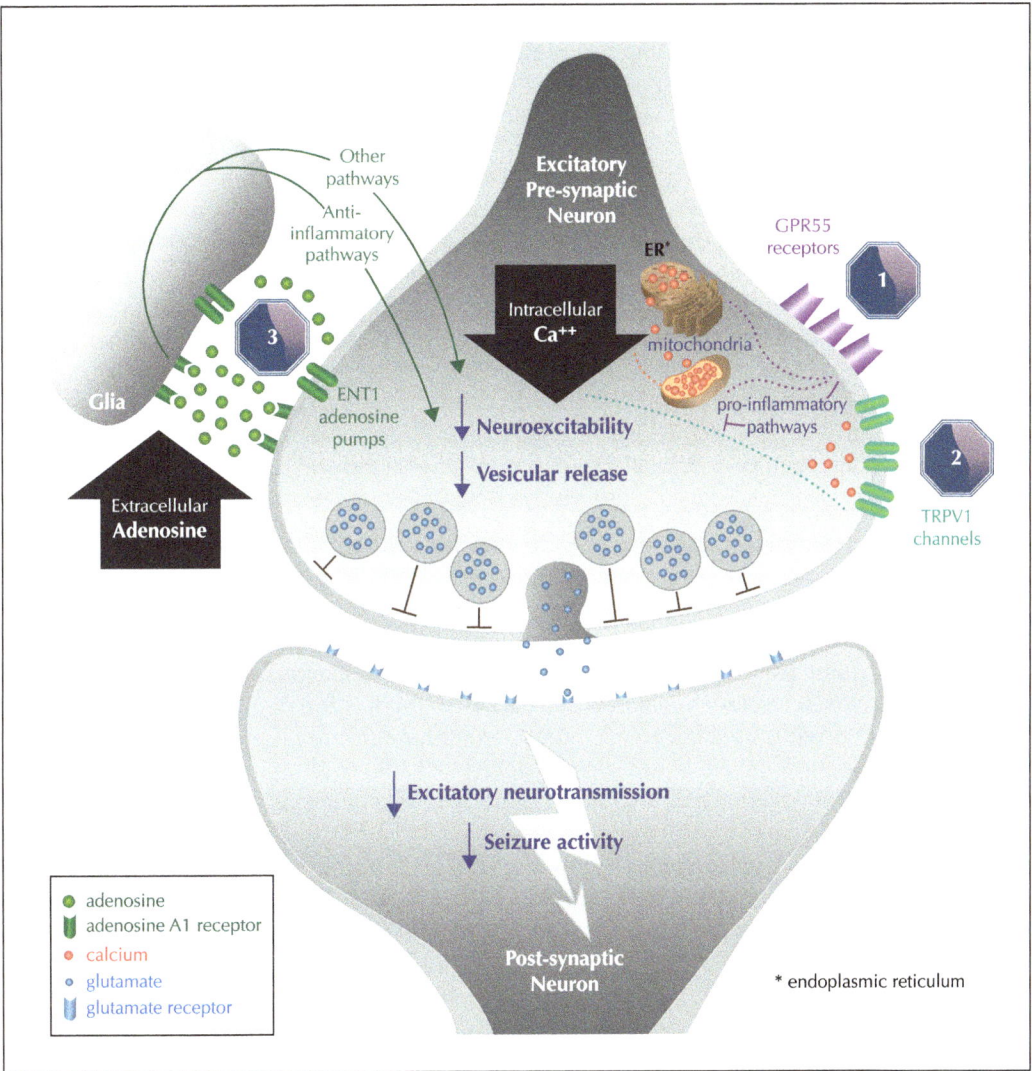

Figure 1/ Proposed multimodal mechanism of action of CBD in epilepsy.

receptors, which upon activation by locally released adenosine, mediate the inhibition of presynaptic calcium influx, and postsynaptic hyperpolarisation through enhancement of inwardly rectifying potassium channels (Fredholm et al., 2005). In addition to the global inhibitory tone conferred by A_1 receptor activation, adenosine further fine tunes neuromodulation, in part, by heterodimerization with other G-protein-coupled receptors and affects all major neurotransmitter and neurotrophin systems (Sebastiao and Ribeiro, 2009).

Adenosine is a well-characterized endogenous anticonvulsant and seizure terminator of the brain through agonism of A_1 and A_{2A} receptors, respectively. While an anti-inflammatory mechanism for seizure control through agonism of A_{2a} receptors has been proposed (Sesbastiao et al., 2000; Ribeiro et al., 2012; Amorim, 2016), a causal link between regulation of neuroinflammation and seizure has not been demonstrated. Therefore, it is yet to be proven that agonism of A_{2a} receptors is implicated in the control of seizure, preventing instigation of neuroinflammatory processes or visa-versa. Endogenous adenosine is uniquely able to control neuronal excitability on multiple levels, and, consequently, any pathological disruption of adenosine homeostasis is likely to affect network excitability. Evidence for the role of adenosine in seizure can be categorised in terms of effects of maladaptive changes in adenosine metabolism observed in epilepsy and the effect of selective pharmacological tools. Maladaptive changes in adenosine metabolism due to increased expression of the astroglial enzyme, adenosine kinase (ADK), play a major role in epileptogenesis (Bioson, 2016). Increased expression of ADK has dual roles in both reducing the inhibitory tone of adenosine in the brain, which consequently reduces the threshold for seizure generation. This process also drives an increased flux of methyl groups through the transmethylation pathway, thereby increasing global DNA methylation (Weltha et al., 2018). Through these mechanisms, adenosine is uniquely positioned to link metabolism with epigenetic outcome. Therapeutic adenosine augmentation therefore is not only central to suppression of seizures in epilepsy, but possibly also to the prevention of epilepsy and its progression overall.

Regarding the mechanism of action of CBD and interaction with the purinergic system, although lacking appreciable affinity for, and agonist activity at either A_1 or A_{2a} receptors, CBD increases extracellular adenosine as exemplified by the effects observed in the rat nucleus accumbens for two hours post-intrahippocampal injection (Mijangos-Moreno et al., 2014). Furthermore, CBD inhibits adenosine uptake into macrophages and microglia by the equilibrative nucleoside transporter and enhances suppression of tumour necrosis factor alpha (TNFα) (Liou et al., 2008). The most compelling direct evidence for CBD's inhibition of adenosine reuptake comes from the ability of CBD to inhibit adenosine transport in rat synaptosomes. Here, CBD maximally inhibited [^{3}H] adenosine uptake into rat synaptosomes in a concentration-dependent manner (IC_{50} 1.1 µM) and the prototypic positive control equilibrative nucleoside transporter-1 (ENT-1) inhibitor dipyridamole exhibited the expected potency (Nichol et al., 2018). The role of adenosine in neuromodulation (Boison et al., 2016) in addition to CBD's effect on adenosine reuptake, suggests that a component of CBD's mechanism of action in seizure control in Dravet and Lennox-Gastaut syndromes is enhancement of adenosine-mediated signalling through increased availability of extracellular adenosine for agonism of A_1 and possibly other centrally-expressed adenosine receptors.

TRPV1 is expressed widely throughout the central nervous system and peripheral afferent fibres (Caterina et al., 1997; Chung et al., 1985; Roberts et al., 2004; Tóth et al., 2005). TRPV1 promotes neuronal depolarization, increasing their firing rate and synaptic activity (Xing and Li, 2007). TRPV1 can be activated by a number of endogenous and exogenous stimuli including heat, N-acyl amides, arachidonic acid (AA) derivatives, vanilloids, protons, and cannabinoids (De Petrocellis et al., 2017). Initial observations by Bisogno and colleagues (2001) describing CBD as a TRPV1 receptor agonist were confirmed by De Petrocellis et al. (2011) who also observed rapid desensitization of the TRPV1 channel following CBD application.

TRPV1 expression is increased in human epilepsy (Sun et al., 2013) and unsurprisingly plays role in regulation of cortical excitability (Mori et al., 2012). The role of TRPV1 in the mechanism of antiepileptic activity of CBD is based upon the observations that CBD can activate and rapidly desensitize TRPV1 receptors at low micromolar concentrations in recombinant systems and in *in vitro* experimental models of epileptiform activity (Iannotti et al., 2014). Here, patch clamp analysis in human TRPV1-transfected HEK293 cells demonstrated that CBD activates and rapidly desensitizes TRPV1 in a concentration-dependent manner and the TRPV1 receptor specificity of the CBD effect confirmed by sensitivity of effect the TRPV1 receptor antagonist, capsazepine.

Moreover, in a recent pivotal study (Gray et al., 2019), the efficacy and potency of CBD on seizure threshold in an acute model of generalized seizure was examined in the TRPV1 knock-out mouse and compared to wild-type litter mates. While CBD dose-dependently increased the current required to induce seizures in 50% of animals, deletion of the *TPRV1* gene resulted in a blunted response to CBD, identifying TRPV1 as a key target implicated in the mechanism of anticonvulsive action of CBD.

In addition to the description of proposed mechanisms of action responsible for the efficacy of CBD against seizures, it is equally important to understand those mechanisms that lack plausibility given the concentrations at which pharmacological engagement is observed. The aetiology of a significant proportion of patients diagnosed with Dravet is a loss of function polymorphism in the *SCN1A* gene. Voltage-gated sodium channel (Na_v) blocking agents used in the treatment of seizures in Dravet Syndrome lack the potential to ameliorate and may exacerbate seizures. While a single report described the modulation of resurgent Na_v current by CBD (Patel et al., 2016) and another described the inhibition of Na_v channel function at concentrations higher than clinically relevant (Ghovanloo et al., 2018), the lack of effect of purified CBD on peak transient current and lack of use-dependent block has been reported (Gray et al., 2017). Similarly, while the positive allosteric modulation of $GABA_A$ chloride current by CBD has been described in recombinant systems (Bakas et al., 2017), this observation has not been independently confirmed and is observed at CBD concentrations in excess of those observed in patients.

While the precise mechanism of action of CBD in humans remains unknown, and there exist several plausible targets engaged by CBD beyond those described here, the preclinical evidence presented strongly implicates three molecular targets in the anticonvulsive properties of CBD. Thus, CBD reduces neuronal excitability through functional antagonism of GPR55 receptors, desensitization of TRPV1 receptors and inhibition of adenosine transport.

Pharmacology and drug interactions of cannabinoids

Cecilie Johannessen Landmark, Ulrich Brandl

■ Pharmacokinetic properties of CBD

CBD has challenging pharmacokinetic properties that differ from most other antiepileptic drugs (AEDs). An ideal drug would have near absolute bioavailability, distribution with low protein binding, and non-CYP mediated metabolism such that elimination would be predictable. In contrast, CBD has limited and variable bioavailability for oral oil formulations (<6%), due to extensive first pass metabolism in the liver (Bialer *et al.*, 2017, 2018). It was recently demonstrated that the absorption is increased 4-5-fold when ingested with a fat-rich meal (Taylor *et al.*, 2018). With new nanotechnology (PTL401 capsules), the relative oral bioavailability of cannabinoids, CBD and tetrahydrocannabidiol (THC), was increased by 31% and 16%, respectively, when compared to oromucosal spray in 14 volunteers (Atsmon *et al.*, 2018).

CBD has a 99 % protein binding capability, leaving only 1% accessible to be distributed across the blood-brain barrier for pharmacological action (*table 1*). Changes in protein binding due to low albumin or interactions with other highly bound drugs could then affect this parameter. The volume of distribution of such drugs is extremely large, and clearance could be affected if the drug is a low extraction drug in the liver. CBD is metabolised through CYP2C19 to the active metabolite, 7-hydroxy-CBD, and further to inactive metabolites as a carboxylic acid and glucuronoids through CYP3A4 and UGTs (*figure 1*). The inactive metabolites are excreted in the faeces and urine (*figure 1*, *table 1*).

Despite the publication of almost 800 articles, revealed in a recent update on the pharmacokinetics of cannabidiol in humans, appropriate data to draw quantitative comparisons was only available from 24 studies (Millar *et al.*, 2018). This highlights the need for more research and documentation.

■ Pharmacokinetic interactions

CBD exhibits numerous interactions with AEDs, both pharmacodynamic and pharmacokinetic (Johannessen Landmark and Patsalos, 2010; Johannessen and Johannessen Landmark, 2010; Johannessen Landmark *et al.*, 2012, 2016; Patsalos, 2013a, 2013b). Pharmacokinetic interactions are easier to evaluate, as the consequence of such interactions includes a change in the serum concentration of the affected drug. Pharmacokinetic interactions may affect the processes of absorption, distribution (protein binding), metabolism, and excretion; the most important step being metabolism by enzyme induction or enzyme inhibition. Commonly used AEDs that interact with CBD include both potent enzyme inducers,

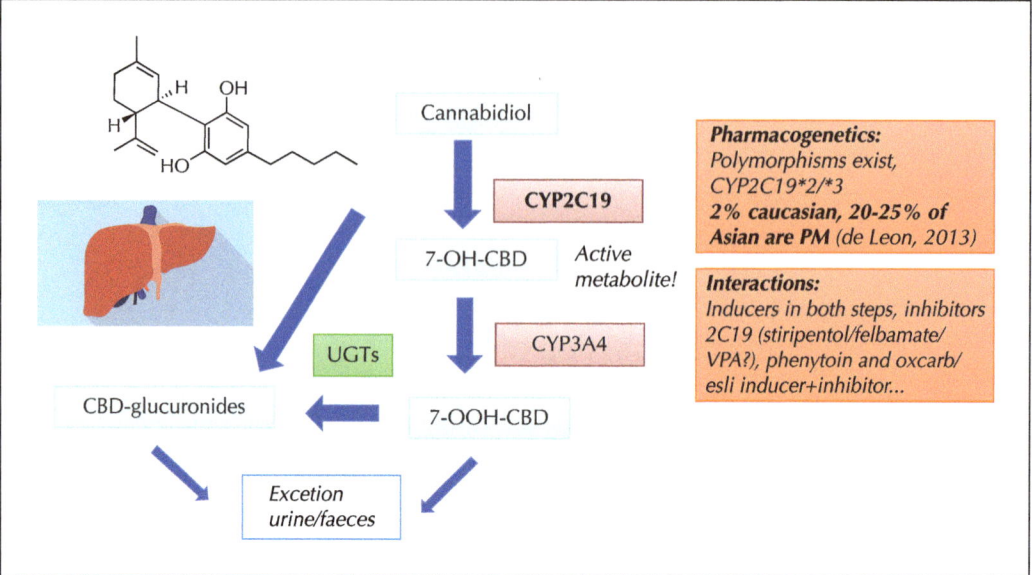

Figure 1/ Metabolism of CBD.
The metabolism of CBD via CYP and UGT enzymes is illustrated; 7-hydroxy-CBD (7-OH-CBD) is an active metabolite, while the carboxylic acid (7-OOH-CBD) is regarded as an inactive metabolite.

Table 1. Pharmacokinetic characteristics of CBD

Pharmacokinetic properties	Comments
Absorption Bioavailability ≈6%, T_{max} 90-120 min, oral oil formulation	Minimal absorption Extensive first-pass metabolism through CYP3A4 Substantial variability between patients, >4-5-fold with a fat-rich meal
Distribution Protein binding 94-99%, V_d 20-40.000 L!	Variability in free fraction? Displacement interactions?
Metabolism CYP3A4, 2C19, UGT1A7,1A9,2B7, $t_{1/2}$ 24-60 h	Strong enzyme-inhibiting properties, PGP?, active metabolite, 7-OH-CBD
Excretion Faeces, urine unchanged 12%	

such as carbamazepine and phenytoin, and inhibitors, such as stiripentol, felbamate, and valproate (Johannessen and Johannessen Landmark, 2010; Johannessen Landmark et al., 2012, 2016; Patsalos, 2013a, 2013b). CBD is also included among the enzyme inhibitors, as illustrated in *figure 2*. The clinical impact of such interactions in the individual patient is difficult to predict and may have no, moderate, or serious consequences. The measurement of unbound CBD concentration in patients would improve our understanding of drug exposure in the body. Patients should be systematically questioned regarding efficacy, tolerability, and adherence, and serum concentrations should be measured and dosages adjusted accordingly, in order to optimize treatment in each patient.

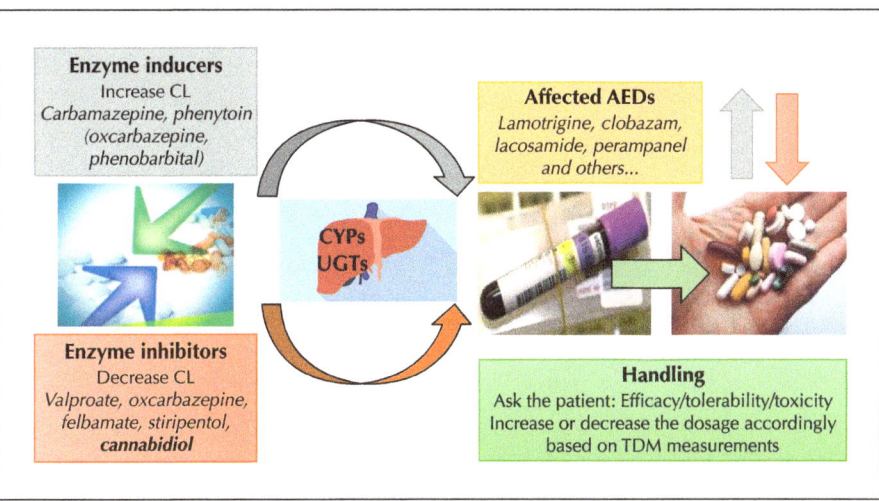

Figure 2/ Pharmacokinetic interactions with AEDs.
Pharmacokinetic interactions with AEDs in the liver involve enzyme induction; an inducer such as carbamazepine or phenytoin speeds up the metabolism of other drugs (such as lamotrigine) by inducing the synthesis of more enzymes. This process often takes a couple of weeks. The result is that the serum concentration of the affected drug is decreased and a dosage adjustment may be needed. The opposite occurs with an enzyme inhibitor, but this process is more rapid as it is only dependent on the half-life of the drugs involved. The serum concentration of the affected drug is increased, and the dosage may then be decreased accordingly, dependent on the serum concentration achieved through therapeutic drug monitoring (TDM). CL: clearance.

■ What do we know so far?

A few studies have characterized the pharmacokinetic interactions between CBD and other concomitantly used drugs, based on the results from clinical trials. Enzyme inhibition by CBD, causing higher levels of various other AEDs, has been shown. Interactions caused by other cannabinoids are less described. The best characterized interaction is the combination of CBD and clobazam, which was a common combination in the clinical studies of CBD. High levels, with up to a five-fold increase in desmethylclobazam, caused an increased risk of toxicity, although there was extensive variability between patients (Geffrey *et al.*, 2015). Sedation was more frequently reported in patients who had high levels of desmethylclobazam (Gaston *et al.*, 2017). This interaction could also contribute to improved seizure control as measured in the studies, however, no comparison of CBD without concomitant use of clobazam has been performed.

Furthermore, serum levels of topiramate, rufinamide, and desmethylclobazam increased moderately in children and adults, and zonisamide and eslicarbazepine levels were found to increase in adults with increasing dose of CBD (Gaston *et al.*, 2017) (*figure 3*). This has to be studied more closely (Franco and Perucca, 2019). The concentration/dose ratio of topiramate increased by 25% in one of our patients in combination with CBD at 20 mg/kg. In addition, we observed a 70% increase in the concentration/dose (C/D) ratio of desmethylclobazam following CBD initiation even at a very low exposure of 1 mg/kg/day (Johannessen Landmark, unpublished observations).

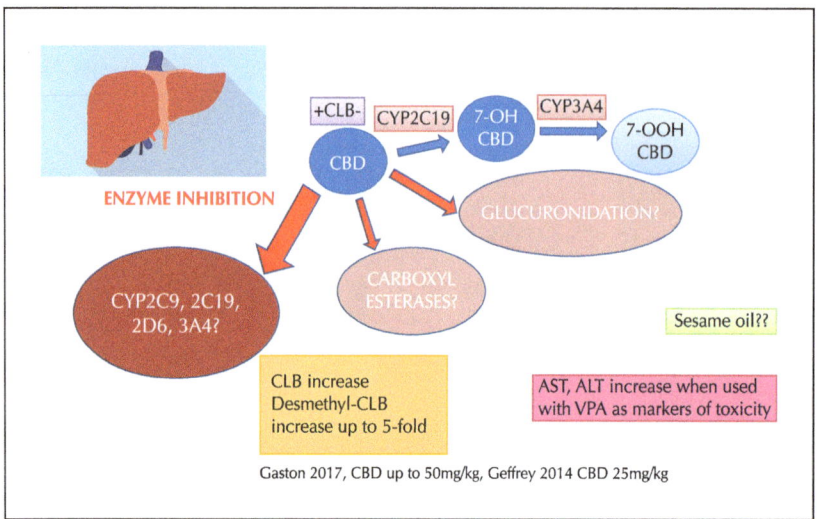

Figure 3/ Pharmacokinetic interactions with CBD.
The pharmacokinetic interactions that have been documented so far are related to metabolism; enzyme inhibition of various CYP and UGT enzymes (Geffrey et al., 2015; Gaston et al., 2017; Bialer et al., 2018; Franco and Perucca, 2019). No interactions regarding protein binding have been identified, however, such interactions are possible based on the high degree of protein binding of CBD as well as other AEDs (valproate, stiripentol).

It is likely that other AEDs would be affected based on their metabolic pathways, and CBD may inhibit drugs such as lamotrigine which is mainly metabolised through UGT1A4 and is highly susceptible to enzyme inducers and inhibitors (Johannessen Landmark and Patsalos, 2010; Johannessen Landmark et al., 2016). Furthermore, anecdotal reports indicate that CBD may influence perampanel, metabolised through CYP3A4, via enzyme inhibition, as increased sleepiness was reported in patients following initiation of CBD.

■ What we do not know?

Possible pharmacokinetic interactions with other AEDs that affect the metabolism of CBD are not yet documented but might be of clinical relevance, such as clobazam. The combination of CBD and stiripentol or valproate is being studied in a Phase 2 trial which may provide answers regarding possible interactions at the level of metabolism as well as protein binding.

Since CBD is metabolised through common pathways that might be affected by other enzyme inducers and inhibitors, conversely, the potential effect of CBD metabolism on other enzyme inducers and inhibitors has not yet been studied. Inducers act at various steps during the metabolism of CBD, CYP3A4, 2C19 and UGTs (carbamazepine, phenytoin), and inhibitors during the metabolism of CYP2C19 and UGTs (stiripentol, felbamate, valproate, and the mixed inducer/inhibitor oxcarbazepine) (Johannessen and Johannessen Landmark, 2010; Patsalos, 2013a; Burns et al., 2016).

Since CBD is 99% protein bound, possible displacement interactions with other highly bound AEDs may occur, such as those commonly used for Dravet syndrome which include stiripentol and valproate. Other candidates might also include clobazam and perampanel based on a recent review of the use of therapeutic drug monitoring (TDM) and measurements of unbound concentrations of all AEDs (Patsalos et al., 2017; Patsalos et al., 2018).

There are therefore still a number of unanswered questions regarding the pharmacology of CBD due to its challenging pharmacokinetics, including absorption and interactions, as also pointed out in a recent expert review (Brodie and Ben-Menachem, 2018).

Recommendations for handling of CBD

Clinical experience has shown that CBD is effective in controlled randomized trials for Dravet and Lennox-Gastaut syndrome. Open drug trials have shown a similar effectiveness in children with CDKL-5, Aicardi syndrome, Dup15q and Doose syndrome (Devinsky et al., 2018a). Many case reports also show successful treatments for other epilepsy syndromes (Arzimanoglou et al., 2020).

CBD is administered orally as an oily solution. In the controlled studies, doses up to 20mg/kg/day were used and in open-label studies even higher doses, mostly up to 25mg/kg, were used. Safety data from the controlled trials show a clear dose dependency of adverse effects such as somnolence, diarrhoea and appetite loss (Devinsky et al., 2018a; Thiele et al., 2018) (figure 4). Most other adverse effects were not significant relative to the placebo groups. The odds ratio for discontinuation due to adverse effects was 1.45 (95% CI: 0.28-7.41; p =0.657) and 4.20 (95% CI: 1.82-9.68; p= 0.001) for CBD at the doses of 10 and 20 mg/kg/day, respectively, in comparison to placebo based on a meta-analysis from the available controlled studies (Lattanzi et al., 2018). Efficacy data, however, show that a significant proportion of children already respond to doses of 10mg/kg/day (figure 4) in studies on Lennox-Gastaut syndrome. Therefore a "start slow" and "increase individually" strategy is recommended. A starting dose of 5mg/kg/day, given in two doses, appears to be adequate.

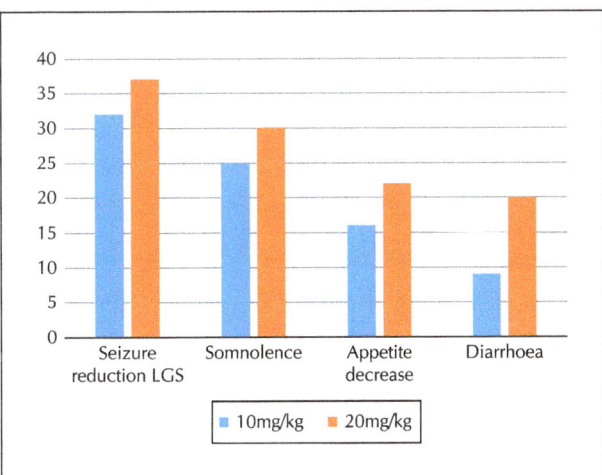

Figure 4/ Dose dependency of efficacy (percentage of seizure reduction; Data pooled from the two controlled Lennox-Gastaut trials 1414 and 1423) and common adverse effects (percentage) at 10 mg/kg and 20 mg/kg CBD. A significant number of patients responded to 10 mg/kg CBD. Adverse effects are clearly dose-dependent. (No efficacy data are available for Dravet syndrome patients treated with 10mg/kg CBD).

> **Box 1. Clinical handling of CBD.**
> - Start low (2.5 or 5 mg/kg/day), increase to 10mg/kg/day after two weeks
> - Review clinical response and adverse effects on 10 mg/kg/day
> - Remain on this dose if effective
> - Otherwise increase dose in steps of 5mg/kg/day if CBD is well tolerated
> - Stop at 20-25mg/kg/day - withdraw CBD if ineffective

This dose should be increased to 10mg/kg/day after two weeks of treatment. Thereafter, the individual response should be carefully observed. The observation time needed strictly depends on baseline seizure frequency before administration of CBD. If the drug is well tolerated but not sufficiently effective, the dose should be slowly increased in increments of 5mg/kg/day, as long as it is tolerated, up to a maximum of 20-25mg/kg/day (box 1).

Handling CBD in combination with clobazam and/or stiripentol

Special care should be taken if CBD is added to clobazam treatment. In some cases, extreme increases in clobazam/desmethylclobazam levels were observed (Devinsky et al., 2018a, 2018b, 2018c). Adverse effects such as fatigue, somnolence, ataxia, a decrease in cognitive function or behavioural changes might indicate toxic benzodiazepine levels. Clinically, this is difficult to distinguish from possible adverse effects of CBD itself. Therefore, monitoring of clobazam/desmethylclobazam levels is strictly recommended. Baseline TDM should be performed in these patients before administration of CBD and then after each increase. If a significant increase in benzodiazepine levels is observed, an adequate decrease in clobazam dose is recommended. Regarding the extent of decrease in dose, an estimate based on linear kinetics is adequate (benzodiazepine levels should be rechecked after dose reduction).

Stiripentol, like CBD, inhibits the same CYP P450 subtype 2C19. Therefore, a further increase in benzodiazepine levels will be uncommon if the patient is already on stiripentol. As the number of available data on these combinations is still limited, it cannot be fully excluded that some patients still might react with a further benzodiazepine increase. This might be the case particularly in patients receiving lower than recommended (50mg/kg/day) doses of stiripentol. Therefore, a baseline clobazam/desmethylclobazam level should also be measured in this patient group. The levels should be re-checked in the event of one of the above-mentioned adverse effects.

Recommendations for drug level and safety monitoring

Regarding safety aspects and risks, the levels of liver enzymes, AST and ALT (markers of toxicity), increased up to more than three-fold in patients who used valproate concomitantly, causing withdrawal of CBD in some cases (Gaston et al., 2017; Devinsky et al., 2018b). In addition to TDM, biochemical markers of toxicity may be measured, such as liver enzymes, for improved knowledge and patient safety (Johannessen Landmark and Johannessen, 2012).

CBD is initially metabolised by CYP2C19, an enzyme that exerts pharmacogenetic variability, and some patients are poor or extra-rapid metabolisers (de Leon et al., 2013;

Johannessen Landmark et al., 2016). Polymorphisms (*1,2,3) exist and are present at different frequencies according to ethnic group; e.g. 2% in Caucasians but 20-25% in the Asian population (de Leon et al., 2013). Thus, pharmacogenetic variability and the possibility that some patients may experience adverse effects at low exposures should be considered. In this regard, previous observations of unexpected high levels of desmethylclobazam should be noted.

The metabolism of CBD has been hypothesised to account for possible CBD-related hepatotoxic effects. In one study, it was shown that 50% of CBD metabolism gave rise to the metabolite, 7-OOH-CBD, which exhibits, in part, the chemical structure of the fatty acid valproate, 2-n-VPA, and this valproate metabolite has been associated with hepatotoxicity as well as teratotogenic effects (Ujvary and Hanus, 2016). One may therefore speculate whether this metabolite of CBD causes the hepatoxic effects by the same mechanism as that involved in valproate-induced hepatotoxicity, however, this remains to be investigated.

Attention to clinical pharmacology and AED interactions, as well as TDM, should reveal these effects and it is highly recommended to follow changes in serum concentrations of all drugs in use for all patients initiating CBD as a basis for appropriate dosage adjustment in order to take this safety aspect into account. TDM should always be requested on clinical grounds and should form the basis for establishing an individual reference range where the patient has achieved an optimal balance between efficacy and tolerability. This concentration would then serve as a reference for further follow-up, dosage adjustments, and initiation and withdrawal of various comedications (Patsalos et al., 2008; Johannessen Landmark et al., 2016; Patsalos et al., 2018). The serum concentrations of other concomitantly used AEDs as well as other relevant drugs in use, such as psychotropic drugs (mood stabilisers, antidepressants, and antipsychotics), should also be followed to reveal possible pharmacokinetic interactions or reasons for poor clinical effects or observed adverse effects.

Pharmacogenetic testing of CYP2C19 could be performed if a poor metabolizer (PM) genotype is suspected based on unexpectedly high levels of CBD relative to the dose.

Safety monitoring of liver enzymes is highly recommended. In the controlled trials, 8% of the patients showed significantly increased liver enzymes at 10 mg/kg/day and 16% at 20mg/kg/day in combination with valproate (Devinsky et al., 2018b). This condition led to withdrawal of CBD if AST or ALT showed a three-fold increase over baseline in the presence of any symptoms (fever, rash, nausea, abdominal pain, or increased bilirubin) or an eight-fold increase in the absence of such symptoms. In rare cases, an increase in ALT/AST was observed with 20mg/kg/day CBD without concomitant use of valproate, but not with lower doses of CBD. The increase in liver enzymes was reversible in about half the cases, without taking any action; in the remaining cases, CBD was withdrawn, leading to normalization of AST/ALT (Devinsky et al., 2018b).

With the exception of clinical trials, significantly increased liver enzymes should lead to at least withdrawal or a reduction of CBD or valproate. A decrease in valproate should be considered first if the patient's history does not indicate a significant benefit with valproate but a favourable effect with the addition of CBD. In all other cases, CBD should be withdrawn or reduced to 10mg/kg. A mild increase in ALT/AST can be observed for a few weeks before taking any action.

■ Conclusions

AEDs exhibit extensive pharmacological variability with numerous interactions with CBD. CBD demonstrates a challenging pharmacokinetic profile with low bioavailability, significant protein binding, and interactions with various metabolic pathways in the liver, including CYPs that are susceptible to pharmacogenetic variability and drug interactions.

More pharmacokinetic studies are needed, as many AEDs are affected, causing increased concentrations and risk of toxicity. The interaction with clobazam has been best characterised, giving rise to a several-fold increase in the active metabolite desmethylclobazam, with risk of excessive adverse effects. Serum concentration measurements and the use of TDM and biochemical markers of toxicity, such as liver enzymes, are important for improved knowledge and patient safety. This is recommended for all patients initiating CBD treatment in order to follow changes in serum concentration of all drugs as a basis for appropriate dosage adjustment.

Since the pharmacokinetics of CBD is highly variable and unpredictive, CBD is used as polytherapy in patients with refractory epilepsy, often with a high drug burden. As there are numerous possible pharmacokinetic interactions resulting in possible toxicity, TDM should be implemented to individualise treatment with CBD, thus pharmacological observations may be documented and related to clinical outcome of CBD treatment in a safe way.

The role of cannabinoids in epilepsy treatment: a critical review of efficacy results from clinical trials

Rima Nabbout, Elizabeth A. Thiele

The use of natural cannabinoids in the treatment of epilepsy was reported in ancient Greek and Arabic medical texts. During the 1850s and 60s there were numerous reports in the medical literature describing the effectiveness of cannabis in the treatment of several medical conditions, including epilepsy. In the 1980s and 90s, several reports of small series or case reports of the use of cannabis extracts in epilepsy yielded contradictory results (Cunha et al., 1980; Ames and Cridland, 1986; Trembly and Sherman, 1990). More recent reports of the efficacy of cannabis use in patients with epilepsy have also been inconclusive (Gross et al., 2004; Hamerle et al., 2014). A limitation of all of these studies was that the composition of the extracts used was not available, and likely highly variable including the concentrations of CBD in the extracts. However, CBD was shown to have anti-seizure activity based on *in vitro* and *in vivo* models (Jones et al., 2010; Devinsky et al., 2014).

A new interest in the clinical use of CBD enriched cannabis extracts in the treatment of pharmacoresistant epilepsies was prompted by media reports of efficacy in children with Dravet syndrome (DS) and surveys of parental evaluation of CBD efficacy from Colorado, USA, where medical cannabis was available for medical prescriptions (Porter and Jacobson, 2013).

In 2013, the first Phase 1 trial for a purified form of CBD (Epidiolex; >99% CBD), developed by GW Pharma, was initiated. Subsequently, a comprehensive program on the efficacy and tolerability of this compound for the treatment of drug-resistant epilepsies was initiated. Results of these trials led to the FDA approval of this formulation of purified CBD on June 25, 2018: *"Epidiolex is indicated for the treatment of seizures associated with Lennox-Gastaut syndrome (LGS) or DS in patients two years of age and older"*. Thus, CBD became the first FDA-approved purified drug substance derived from cannabis and also the first FDA-approved drug for the treatment of seizures in DS. More recently, Epidyolex was also approved by the European Medicines Agency as treatment for DS and LGS in combination with clobazam treatment.

This chapter will detail the clinical studies using purified CBD (Epidiolex), including the first open interventional exploratory study and RCTs for DS and LGS:

- Drug-resistant epilepsy in childhood and young adults (2-30 years old): an expanded access program in the USA (Devinsky et al., 2016);
- Dravet syndrome: two RCTs (GWCARE 1 et 2) (Devinsky et al., 2017);
- Lennox-Gastaut syndrome: two RCTs (GWCARE 3 and 4) (Thiele et al., 2018; Devinsky et al., 2018a);
- Dravet syndrome: an open-label extension study (GWCARE 5) (Devinsky et al., 2019).

■ Prospective open interventional study (Devinsky et al., 2016)

This open-label interventional trial recruited children and young adults with drug-resistant, childhood-onset epilepsies. This design was organized as a large exploratory study in patients with drug-resistant epilepsies fulfilling the following inclusion criteria: age 1-30 years, pharmacoresistant childhood-onset epilepsy, more than four countable seizures with a motor component over a four-week period, and a stable therapy regimen (AEDs, ketogenic diet, VNS) for at least four weeks prior to enrolment.

After enrolment, patients had a four-week baseline period in which parents kept a seizure diary. After this observational period, Epidiolex was added to the patients' current regimen at 2-5mg/kg/d, divided twice daily, then increased by 2-5mg/kg/d every week until intolerance or until a dose of 25-50mg/kg/d was reached.

The primary objective was to establish the safety and tolerability of CBD, and the primary efficacy endpoint was median percentage change in the mean monthly frequency of motor seizures at 12 weeks. Efficacy was examined based on modified intention-to-treat analysis.

Between January 15, 2014, and January 15, 2015, 214 patients were enrolled; 162 (76%) patients who had at least 12 weeks of follow-up after the first dose of CBD were included in the safety and tolerability analysis, and 137 (64%) patients were included in the efficacy analysis.

In the safety group, 33 (20%) patients had DS and 31 (19%) patients had LGS. The remaining patients had different drug-resistant epilepsies with variable syndromes and aetiologies including patients with *CDKL5* mutations, tuberous sclerosis complex, and myoclonic atonic epilepsy.

Tolerability and safety data were obtained for 162 patients (76%). Of this group, 78% showed adverse events (AEs), with somnolence in 25%, decreased appetite in 19%, diarrhoea in 19%, and fatigue in 13%. Serious AEs were reported in 20%, with status epilepticus, diarrhoea, and weight loss being the most common. Serious AEs (status epilepticus and diarrhoea plus weight loss) led to treatment discontinuation in 3% of patients.

For the efficacy analysis, the median reduction of motor seizures reached 36.5% over the 12-week treatment period, with five patients free of motor seizures. Reduction was >50% in 39%, >70% in 21%, and >90% in 9%. The median reduction was higher for patients with DS, who reached 49.8% reduction. Patients with atonic seizures (32 patients) showed a significant response, as 56% had >50% reduction in seizures and 16% became seizure-free (Devinsky et al., 2016).

■ Dravet syndrome (DS)

DS is an infantile-onset epilepsy presenting in a previously normal child before the age of 15 months (and often before one year of age) with prolonged, typically febrile and hemiclonic, seizures evolving into status epilepticus. Patients progressively develop other seizure types a few months after the onset including myoclonic, focal, and generalized tonic-clonic seizures, accompanied by developmental plateauing. DS is a highly pharmacoresistant epilepsy with poor developmental outcome including psychiatric disorders and disorders of behaviour, gait, sleep, and speech.

Prior to these trials, only one drug had completed a RCT for DS during its development (Diacomit*, Biocodex) and was registered in Europe in 2014 and in the USA in 2019, in association with clobazam. Other drugs showed variable degrees of efficacy on seizure reduction in patients with DS but were reported mostly in retrospective studies, and less in prospective studies. These treatments included topiramate, zonisamide, the ketogenic diet, and bromide. The treatment approach in different countries varies depending upon medication availability. Patients with DS are usually on polytherapy and seizure control is rarely achieved (De Liso *et al*., 2016). Thirty-two patients with DS were included in the first open-label CBD interventional trial; as described above, patients with DS showed a median decrease in motor seizures of 49.8% showing a higher response in this group compared to 36.5% median reduction of motor seizures in the trial at large, over the 12-week treatment period. This exploratory study provided a promising "signal" (Chiron *et al*., 2013) to continue further development of CBD for patients with DS and LGS.

Randomized controlled trial for DS (GWPCARE1) (Devinsky *et al*., 2017)

This study included patients with DS aged two to 18 years, with confirmation of a diagnosis made by the epilepsy study consortium. For eligibility, patients had to be inadequately controlled by at least one current drug and have ≥four convulsive seizures (tonic-clonic, tonic, clonic, or atonic seizures) during the four-week baseline period.

Exclusion criteria included: use of any other cannabis derivative within three months prior to entering or during the study, presence of a progressive diagnosed medical illness, evidence of impaired hepatic function on laboratory testing, and known or suspected hypersensitivity to cannabinoids or any of the excipients of the investigational medicinal products.

CBD oral solution (100mg/ml) or placebo was added to current AEDs starting at 2.5mg/kg/day and titrated to 20mg/kg/day over two weeks. The dose of 20mg/kg/d was set by an independent drug safety monitoring committee based on pharmacokinetic and safety data from an initial part of this study (Part A) evaluating doses of 5, 10, and 20mg/kg/day. The titration period was followed by a 12-week dose-maintenance period. The total treatment duration was 14 weeks, comprising the two-week titration period plus the 12-week treatment period.

The primary endpoint was the median percentage change in convulsive seizure frequency from the four-week baseline period compared to the 14-week treatment period among patients who received CBD, compared with placebo. The secondary endpoint measures included: the Caregiver Global Impression of Change (CGIC), assessed on a Likert-like scale; the number of patients with at least 25%, 50%, 75% and 100% reduction in convulsive seizure frequency; the duration of seizure subtypes assessed by the caregiver (decrease, no change, or increase in average duration); sleep disruption, assessed on a numerical rating scale from 0 to 10; the change in score on the Epworth Sleepiness Scale; score based on the Quality of Life in Childhood Epilepsy questionnaire; score based on the Vineland Adaptive Behaviour Scales (second edition); the number of hospitalizations due to epilepsy; the number of patients with emergence of new seizures types compared to baseline period; and the use of rescue medication.

The safety profile of CBD was assessed on the basis of the number, type, and severity of AEs as well as the Columbia Suicide Severity Rating Scale (for patients ≥six years of age, when appropriate), vital signs, electrocardiographic variables, laboratory safety variables, and physical examination variables; safety end points were monitored at each visit. The palatability of the trial agent was assessed by caregivers on a 5-point scale, ranging from "liked it a lot" to "did not like it at all".

This study recruited in 33 study centres in the US and Europe. Over all centres, 177 patients were screened and 120 were randomized. The median age at inclusion was 9.7 years (range: 2.5-18.0) in the CBD group and 9.8 years (range: 2.3-18.4) in the placebo group. Patients in both groups had previously been treated with a median of four AEDs (0-26 for the CBD group and 0-14 for the placebo) and were currently on a median of three AEDS (1-5) for both groups. Seizure number in the four-week baseline period did not differ significantly, with 12.4 (6.2-28) seizures in the CBD group and 14.9 (7-36) in the placebo group.

The median reduction in seizure frequency was significantly higher in the CBD group during both the total treatment period (39% *vs.* 13%; $p=0.01$) and maintenance period (41 *vs.* 16%, $p=0.002$). Based on the CGIC scale, 37 of 60 caregivers (62%) judged their child's overall condition to improve in the CBD group, compared with 20 of 58 caregivers (34%) in the placebo group ($p=0.02$). There was no significant difference in sleep scores or QoL scales, moreover, no worsening was reported.

The adverse-event profile of CBD in this trial was similar to that seen in the open-label interventional study, including somnolence (36% in the CBD group *vs.* 10% in the placebo group), loss of appetite (28% *vs.* 5%), and diarrhoea (31% *vs.* 10%). Of the 22 patients in the CBD group in whom somnolence was reported, 18 were taking clobazam, compared with five of six patients in the placebo group. AEs led to a dose reduction in 10 patients in the CBD group, with complete resolution in eight patients and partial resolution in one patient; in the remaining patient, the AE (loss of appetite) was ongoing. There were few dose adjustments of concomitant antiepileptic drugs during the trial. Abnormalities of hepatic aminotransferase levels occurred only in patients taking valproate, and all resolved spontaneously or with a dosage decrease.

Serious AEs were more common in the CBD group than in the placebo group (16% *vs.* 5%), and AEs led to withdrawal in eight patients in the CBD group compared with one in the placebo group.

■ Lennox Gastaut syndrome (LGS)

Randomized controlled trial I for LGS (GWPCARE3) (Thiele *et al.*, 2018)

This RCT included patients aged 2-55 years with a diagnosis of LGS. LGS diagnosis was based on evidence of >one type of generalized seizure, including drop seizures for ≥six months with documented history of a slow (<3-Hz) spike-and-wave pattern on the EEG. Diagnosis was confirmed by the epilepsy study consortium.

Eligibility criteria included: refractory seizures on more than two AEDs, inclusive of previous and current treatment with at least one AED at the time of inclusion; eight or more drop seizures during the four-week baseline period provided that the patient presented with at least two seizures per week; and all medications and interventions for epilepsy (including the ketogenic diet and vagus nerve stimulation) stable for four weeks before screening.

Exclusion criteria were applied for any patient who: used any cannabinoid derivative within three months of entering the study or not abstaining from use during the study; presented a progressive diagnosed medical illnesses; was initially administered felbamate within the past 12 months; showed significantly impaired hepatic function on liver tests; and finally patients with known or suspected hypersensitivity to cannabinoids or any of the excipients of the investigational medicinal products.

CBD oral solution (100mg/ml) or placebo was added to current AEDs starting at 2.5mg/kg/day and titrated to 20mg/kg/day over two weeks. This titration period was followed by a 12-week dose-maintenance period. The overall duration of the treatment period was 14 weeks; two weeks titration plus the 12 weeks of treatment.

The primary end point was the percentage of change from baseline in drop seizures over the 14-week treatment period. The secondary endpoints included the proportion of patients achieving a >50% reduction in drop seizures, the percentage of change in total seizure frequency, and finally the change from baseline in patient and caregiver global impression of change.

In this study, 171 patients were randomized (86 to CBD and 85 to placebo). The mean age was 15 years with 34% over 18 years. Patients included had previously tried a median of six AEDs and were currently taking a median of three. The median drop seizure frequency over the four-week baseline was 74.

During the 14-week treatment period, patients on CBD achieved a 44% median reduction in drop seizure frequency *vs.* 22% in the placebo group (primary end point; $p=0.0135$). In the same treatment period, patients had a 49% median reduction in non-drop seizures *vs.* 23% in the placebo group ($p=0.004$). Regarding the response for both seizure types (drop and non-drop), patients on CBD had a 41.2% median reduction in seizure frequency compared to 13.7% in the placebo group ($p=0.0005$).

In addition to seizure frequency reduction, in the CBD group, caregivers or patients were significantly more likely to report an improvement in condition (OR=2.54 ; $p=0.0012$).

A total of 86% patients in the CBD and 69% in the placebo group had AEs, with 78% rated as mild or moderate in the CBD group. The major treatment-emergent AEs were diarrhoea, somnolence, pyrexia, and decreased appetite.

A higher incidence of somnolence was observed in patients on AED regimens that included clobazam (CLB) compared with those without CLB for both the CBD (22% *vs.* 9% patients) and placebo (16% *vs.* 2% of patients) groups. In addition, in the CBD group, a higher incidence of elevated transaminases was observed in patients on antiepileptic drug regimens that included valproate compared to those without valproate (19% *vs.* 5%).

Randomized controlled trial 2 for LGS (GWPCARE4) (Devinsky et al., 2018a)

This RCT was designed with the same inclusion and exclusion criteria as well as primary and secondary endpoints and the first LGS trial. The only difference with the previous study was the addition of a third arm consisting of CBD at a lower dose of 10mg/kg/d.

A total of 225 patients were randomized; 76 to 20mg/kg/day, 73 to 10mg/kg/day, and 76 to placebo. The mean age was 15.3 (2.6-43.4 for the placebo group, and 15.4 [2.6-42.6] and 16 years [2.6-48] for the 10 and 20 mg/kg/day CBD groups, respectively). The number of drop seizures during the four-week baseline was 80.3 (47.8-148.0), 86.9 (40.6-190.0), and 85.5 (38.3-161.5) in the 20mg/kg/d, 10mg/kg/d, and placebo group, respectively.

The reduction in seizure frequency was 41.9% and 37.2% in the 20 and 10mg/kg/d CBD group, respectively, vs. 17.2% in the placebo group, revealing a significant difference in both CBD arms relative to placebo ($p=0.005$ and $p=0.002$, respectively).

Somnolence, diarrhoea, and decreased appetite were the major treatment-emergent AEs. An increase in liver enzymes was predominantly found in patients with valproate.

Open-label extension study (GWPCARE5) (Devinsky et al., 2019)

Patients who completed GWPCARE1 Part A (NCT02091206) or Part B, or a second placebo-controlled trial, GWPCARE2 (NCT02224703) (data not published), were invited to enroll in a long-term open-label extension trial, GWPCARE5 (NCT02224573). GWP-CARE5 is an ongoing open-label extension trial of add-on CBD in patients with DS who completed GWPCARE1 or GWPCARE2 and patients with LGS who completed treatment in one of two Phase 3 trials (GWPCARE 3 and GWPCARE4).

The first report of GWPCARE5 is the interim analysis for safety, efficacy, and patient-reported outcomes for patients with DS enrolled in this open study (Devinsky et al., 2019).

Patients entered this extension phase after the end of the maintenance period of 12 weeks. Investigators could decrease the dose of CBD and/or concomitant AEDs if a patient experienced intolerance or could increase the dose to a maximum of 30mg/kg/d if thought to be of benefit by the physician. The data cut-off for this interim analysis was November 3, 2016.

The primary objective of this open-label extension was to evaluate the long-term safety and tolerability of adjunctive CBD treatment, based on treatment-emergent AEs (occurring at any time during the open-label extension, from enrolment through to follow-up visit), vital signs, 12-lead electrocardiograms, and clinical laboratory parameters. Secondary objectives were to evaluate the efficacy of CBD and patient-reported outcomes based on changes in the Subject/Caregiver Global Impression of Change (S/CGIC) scale.

By November 2016, at the time of cut-off analysis for GWPCARE5, 278 patients with DS from the completed GWCARE1 study and the ongoing GWCARE2 study had completed the original randomized trials, and 264 (95%) enrolled in this open-label extension.

Median treatment duration was 274 days (range: 1-512) with a mean modal dose of 21mg/kg/d. Patients received a median of three concomitant antiepileptic medications. AEs occurred in 93.2% of patients and were mostly mild (36.7%) or moderate (39.0%). Commonly reported

AEs were the same as those reported in the RCTs: diarrhoea (34.5%), pyrexia (27.3%), decreased appetite (25.4%), and somnolence (24.6%). Seventeen patients (6.4%) discontinued due to AEs. Twenty-two of 128 patients from GWPCARE1 (17.2%), all on valproic acid, had elevated liver transaminase, ≥three times greater than the upper normal limit.

In patients from GWPCARE1 Part B, median reduction from baseline in monthly seizure frequency, assessed in 12-week periods up to Week 48, ranged from 38% to 44% for convulsive seizures and 39% to 51% for total seizures. After 48 weeks of treatment, 85% of patients/caregivers reported improvement in the patients' overall condition based on the Subject/Caregiver Global Impression of Change scale.

This trial showed a good tolerance of long-term CBD treatment with an acceptable safety profile without new-emergent side effects. CBD led to a sustained and clinically meaningful reduction in seizure frequency in patients with treatment-resistant DS in this extension phase.

Conclusion

CBD has been shown to be effective, safe, and well tolerated as a treatment for DS and LGS. CBD (20mg/kg/day) as an add-on to existing AEDs resulted in significantly greater reductions in total seizure frequency *vs.* placebo with a significant reduction of convulsive seizures *vs.* add-on placebo in patients with DS and drop seizures in patients with LGS. This efficacy was achieved on 20mg/kg/d in DS and LGS trials but also on 10mg/kg/d in one LGS trial. CBD showed higher efficacy when associated with CLB. This synergy could be at least partially due to an increase in nor-CLB, the active compound of CLB, due an inhibition of Cyp2C19.

CBD treatment resulted in more AEs than placebo. Most common AEs were somnolence, diarrhoea, and decreased appetite. A higher risk of somnolence was associated with the combination of CBD and CLB, requiring dose adjustment (Devinsky *et al.*, 2018b).

Abnormal hepatic aminotransferase levels were identified predominantly in patients taking concomitant valproate, suggesting an interaction in which CBD may potentiate a valproic acid-induced change in hepatic aminotransferase levels. A few patients exited the trial or the open-label extension study due to AEs.

Compared to placebo, caregivers were significantly more likely to report an improvement in overall condition for patients taking CBD, as measured on the CGIC scale.

The CBD expanded access program (Devinsky *et al.*, 2016) suggests that CBD may have a wider spectrum of efficacy beyond DS and LGS. Results from a randomized controlled trial of CBD in refractory epilepsy in tuberous sclerosis complex were recently released and showed similar efficacy and tolerability. These results along with further results from the expanded access program will help to establish the best guidelines for the use of CBD.

Adverse effects of cannabinoids

Carla Anciones, Antonio Gil-Nagel

Cannabis sativa contains more than 80 phytocannabinoids, but little is known about the potential therapeutic effects of most of these molecules. One compound, cannabidiol (CBD) is present at high concentrations in the plant and has demonstrated antiepileptic properties. The medical use of whole-plant cannabis extract is limited by the THC-induced psychoactive properties and the long-term cognitive side effects associated with chronic use (Devinsky, 2016). Safety data published for CBD-containing compounds in adults with different neurological disorders by Koppel *et al.* (2014) was followed by clinical trials, leading to the approval of a high-CBD-concentration oral solution (Epidiolex) for treatment of seizures in patients with Dravet syndrome and Lennox-Gastaut syndrome by the Food and Drug Administration in June 2018 and European Medicines Agency in July 2019.

Short and long-term adverse events of CBD reported in clinical trials

Adverse effects of CBD in patients with treatment-resistant epilepsy are well-documented in randomized and open-label trials. In the first specific double-blinded randomized trial for CBD in children with Dravet syndrome (DS) (Devinsky *et al.*, 2017), adverse events (AEs) were reported in 93% of patients in the CBD group compared to 75% in the placebo group. Most of them (89%) were mild or moderate, appeared in the two-week escalation period, and in two thirds resolved in the first four weeks of treatment. In most patients with DS, the maximal CBD tolerable dose is 20 mg/kg/day (McCoy *et al.*, 2018) and side effects seem to be positively correlated with higher doses of CBD. Most commonly reported CBD AEs include somnolence (22%), diarrhoea (19%), and decreased appetite (17%). Other less frequent AEs include vomiting, fatigue, weight loss, pyrexia, and upper respiratory tract infections. This was consistently found in subsequent clinical trials exploring tolerability of different doses of CBD (Devinsky *et al.*, 2018a, 2018b).

Serious adverse events appear in around 15% of patients treated with CBD. The most significant is the harmful elevation (three times the upper the normal limit) of alanine transaminase (ALT) and aspartate transaminase (AST) levels. Elevation of liver enzymes is also more frequent on high doses of CBD (20 mg/kg/day) and concomitant treatment with valproic acid (Devinsky *et al.*, 2019). Rash has rarely been reported but can appear in association with pyrexia and may lead to discontinuation of the drug (Devinsky *et al.*, 2018a).

When starting a new antiepileptic drug for DS, consideration of the potential pharmacological interactions between given medications is necessary, especially with clobazam (Johannessen Landmark and Brandl, 2020). CBD undergoes significant metabolism via different isoforms of the cytochrome (CYP) P-450 metabolic pathways, CYP 2C9 and 3A4 (Stout and Cimino, 2014), and at the same time constitutes a potent inhibitor of both enzymes. Clobazam metabolism similarly involves CYP 3A4 and in a minor way, CYP 2C19; both of these enzymes catalyse the metabolism of its active metabolite, N-desmetylclobazam (norclobazam; N-CLB) (Geffrey et al., 2015). Uncontrolled studies have shown that the level of N-CLB is increased by CBD, which might lead to a synergistic antiepileptic effect as well as an increase in the rate of AEs in patients taking both drugs, especially somnolence. Phenotypic variability of CYP 2C19 due to polymorphisms can produce variations in N-CLB in patients taking not only CBD but also different antiepileptic drugs that are also metabolic substrates of the CYP-450 pathway. Measurement of serum N-CLB concentrations can be clinically useful for the identification of vulnerable individuals with unexpected moderate and severe AEs (Yamamoto et al., 2013). Surprisingly, elevation of N-CLB in patients taking CBD does not occur in the presence of stiripentol, a strong inhibitor of CYP 2C19, which may interfere with clobazam metabolism (Devinsky et al., 2018a). This is probably explained by normalization of N-CLB levels due to drug dose adjustments prior to the initiation of CBD. There is no apparent significant pharmacokinetic effect between CBD and other concomitant AEDs (valproate, topiramate, levetiracetam, rufinamide, lamotrigine, felbamate or zonisamide) (Gaston et al., 2017).

Most of the AEs in patients with LGS taking CBD are similar to those reported in the DS trials. However, when looking at raw data in the CBD pivotal trials, AEs seem to be more frequent in the DS sample than in LGS. In the study by Devinsky et al. (2018b) for CBD as an add-on treatment for drug-resistant seizures in LGS, three branches of treatment were included: a 20 mg/kg/day group, a 10 mg/kg/day group, and a placebo group. In the 20 mg/kg/day CBD group, several observed adverse events had a similar incidence in both DS and LGS studies: somnolence was observed in 36% *vs.* 30%, decreased appetite in 28% *vs.* 26%, vomiting in 15% *vs.* 12%, and pyrexia in 15% *vs.* 12% in DS and LGS patients, respectively. More strikingly, diarrhoea was more common in DS (31%) than in LGS (13%). This difference may be explained by age differences between both subgroups (2-55 years in the LGS group *vs.* 2-18 years in the DS group), differences in background medications, or, less likely, a disease-specific vulnerability for the drug.

Some very infrequent AEs were reported in patients with LGS taking CBD, such as elevation of γ-glutamyltransferase concentration, increased seizure frequency during weaning-off medication, constipation, and worsening of previous chronic cholecystitis. Elevation of serum transaminases was also a serious adverse event in the pivotal trial, however, none of the patients met the criteria for severe drug-induced liver injury. Most of these AEs occurred within the first 30 days of treatment (Lattanzi et al., 2018) and were reported in patients on high CBD doses as well as valproic acid (Thiele et al., 2018).

Few data are available to assess the safety profile of CBD for epileptic syndromes other than DS and LGS. The first open-label interventional trial for CBD for several types of drug-resistant epilepsy by Devinsky et al. (2016) included a wide heterogeneous group of patients with epilepsy due to different aetiologies (from *CDKL5* mutations or Aicardi syndrome to generalized epilepsies such as Jeavon's syndrome). Post-hoc analysis was made only for patients with DS and LGS difficult to extrapolate to other types of epilepsy (*table 1*). However, in this trial in which doses of CBD were raised up to 50 mg/kg/day, some serious AEs were reported in patients concomitantly taking valproate, such as severe hyperammonaemia that led to CBD discontinuation or severe thrombocytopenia which resolved when valproate was stopped. The relationship between hyperammonaemia and other adverse events has not been systematically assessed in other studies, leaving some areas for improvement in AE identification and management in the future.

Table 1. Adverse events reported by Devinsky *et al.* (2016) based on an open-label study of 214 patients, aged 1-30 years, with drug-resistant epilepsy

	Safety analysis group (*n*=162)
Adverse events (reported in >5 % patients)	
Somnolence	41 (25%)
Decreased appetite	31 (19%)
Diarrhoea	31 (19%)
Fatigue	21 (13%)
Convulsion	18 (11%)
Increased appetite	14 (9%)
Status epilepticus	13 (8%)
Lethargy	12 (7%)
Weight increased	12 (7%)
Weight decreased	10 (6%)
Drug concentration increased	9 (6%)
Treatment-emergent serious adverse events*	
Status epilepticus	9 (6%)
Diarrhoea	3 (2%)
Weight decreased	2 (1%)
Convulsion	1 (<1%)
Decreased appetite	1 (<1%)
Drug concentration increased	1 (<1%)
Hepatotoxicity	1 (<1%)
Hyperammonaemia	1 (<1%)
Lethargy	1 (<1%)
Unspecified pneumonia	1 (<1%)
Aspiration pneumonia	1 (<1%)
Bacterial pneumonia	1 (<1%)
Thrombocytopenia	1 (<1%)

Data are presented as *n* (%). One patient might have had more than one serious adverse event.
* Reported by the investigator to be possibly related to CBD use.

Efficacy of CBD for pharmaco-resistant epilepsy in patients with tuberous sclerosis complex has been studied in a small non-controlled trial of 18 patients in which CBD was added, up to 50 mg/kg/day to their regular antiepileptic therapy (Hess *et al.*, 2016). The most frequent observed AE was drowsiness (44%) followed by ataxia (27.8%) and diarrhoea (22.2%); none of these AEs were considered serious by the investigators. Interestingly, most patients experiencing AEs were taking clobazam and were less likely to reach the high target dose of the study, requiring dose adjustments of either CBD or clobazam to reduce the intensity of the AEs. A small non-placebo, controlled trial to assess the efficacy of CBD in seven paediatric patients with febrile infection-related epilepsy (FIRES) is also documented and reveals mild side effects that include dizziness, decreased appetite, weight loss, and nausea/vomiting (Gofshteyn *et al.*, 2017).

■ Conclusions

Compared to other antiseizure drugs approved for treatment of DS and LGS, more information was available prior to marketing for CBD (Epidiolex/Epidyolex). CBD is generally a well-tolerated drug, with most AEs being mild or moderate and improving either with treatment maintenance or reduction of dosage (Arzimanoglou *et al.*, 2020). The most frequent AEs include somnolence, decreased appetite, and diarrhoea. Most of the side effects occur at the beginning of treatment with doses above 20 mg/kg/day. Prior to starting CBD, a careful assessment of concomitant antiepileptic drugs should be performed, particularly valproic acid, as this combination with CBD is associated with transaminase elevation and decreased platelet count. Also, clobazam, jointly administered with CBD, may produce an increase in somnolence due to nor-clobazam elevation. Additional studies are necessary to identify the reasons for gastrointestinal side effects and provide alternatives to improve the tolerance of CBD in these patients.

Long-term effects of cannabinoids on development/behaviour

Lieven Lagae

With the increased use of cannabis products in young children with epilepsy, it becomes necessary to consider potential negative long-term effects in the developing brain; in particular, special attention should be paid to effects on cognition and behaviour.

It is very well recognized that cannabis use in adolescents and adults can induce negative cognitive and behavioural effects. These effects include problems with concentration and memory, mood changes, and aggressive behaviour which subsequently can lead to, for instance, problems at school, risky sexual behaviour, and more traffic accidents. The "cannabis use disorder", which can be the result of prolonged cannabis use, is described in the DSM-V (American Psychiatry Association, 2013; Gordon et al., 2013). Psychosis, anxiety disorder, and increased suicide risk are part of this chronic disorder. Also, academic and occupational problems are frequently seen in this chronic condition. It is unclear and probably subject-dependent how long and/or how much cannabis is needed to get to the stage of this cannabis use disorder. Most of these negative effects can be explained more by tetrahydrocannabinol (THC) than by cannabidiol (CBD), the two main components of cannabis. The exact cumulative dosage of the individual cannabis components sufficient for the development of cannabis use disorder is not well known. Whether we can expect similar negative effects with the use of medicinal cannabis derivates in young children is not known either. It is reassuring that the products which are now being used in childhood epilepsy contain little THC. However, even with combinations of 95% CBD and 5% THC, substantial amounts of THC are given chronically when one prescribes 10 to 20 mg/kg/day of CBD to try to control the epilepsy. The effect of THC on developing neurons is now relatively clear (Bossong and Niesink, 2010). In normal conditions, the release of excitatory glutamate is fine-tuned by the release of endocannabinoids acting on presynaptic CB1 receptors. This fine regulation actually drives the normal process of pruning in developing neurons. Exogenous THC blocks the presynaptic CB1 receptors thereby disrupting this regulation of neurotransmitter release, with consequent excessive glutamate excitation of the immature NMDA receptor. How much this can affect normal development is a matter of debate. It can be hypothesized indeed that over-exposure to exogenous THC can impact normal learning in early life.

This short review will primarily focus on potential effects on cognition and behaviour associated with early cannabis use. The following three sources of information will be reviewed regarding the study of potential negative long-term effects of cannabis products in the developing brain:

- The recent data obtained from randomized controlled trials (RCTs), examining the effect of treatment on quality of life and adaptive scales. These effects can be considered semi-chronic effects as typical double-blind placebo-controlled trials last for a maximum of 16-20 weeks.
- There is actually a wealth of preclinical and clinical data on the use of cannabis during pregnancy and the effects on the developing brain of the foetus, newborn, and young child.
- Because exposure to recreational cannabis occurs earlier and earlier, studies are now also available on the long-term effects associated with this early adolescent use.

Data from clinical trials

We here refer mainly to the regulatory trials with CBD for Dravet syndrome and Lennox Gastaut syndrome (Devinsky *et al.*, 2017, 2018).

In these trials with cannabidiol (Epidiolex, GW Pharma), the effect of CBD treatment was also measured looking at changes in sleep behaviour, (sleep disruption score, Epworth sleepiness scale score), Quality of Life scores (Quality of Life in Childhood Epilepsy [QOLCE]), and adaptive behaviour (Vineland II). Although there was a positive effect for all parameters studied in the Dravet study, this positive effect was only statistically significant for the Epworth sleepiness score (Devinsky *et al.*, 2017).

Quality of life was measured using the QOLCE; this is composed of 16 subscales which measure changes in physical function, social function, emotional wellbeing, cognition, general health, and general quality of life (Sabaz *et al.*, 2003). In the Lennox Gastaut trial, positive changes were seen in all domains of the QOLCE with actually significant positive changes for language and memory subscales (unpublished results). However, the positive effect on language was only seen in the lower dose arm (10 mg/kg/day). A concern looking at these rather reassuring data is that the QOLCE was administered in less than 30% of the participants. In the Dravet study, more subjects (up to 60%) completed the QOLCE but no statistical differences were seen. It is reassuring that during these trials, no worsening of these important functions was seen.

Overall, behavioural changes were studied using the Vineland Adaptive Behaviour Scales (VABS). The VABS is a commonly used measure of adaptive behaviour skills for children and adolescents up to 18 years of age (Sparrow and Cicchetti, 1985). In addition to providing an overall composite score, it consists of three subscales: (a) communication (receptive, expressive, written); (b) socialization (interpersonal relationships, play and leisure, coping skills); and (c) daily living (person, domestic, community). As for the quality of life scales, no consistent significant changes were seen. In the Lennox Gastaut trial, a small but statistically significant improvement in the socialization domain was seen. In the Dravet trial, a significant improvement was seen in the communication domain, but here only 30% participated in this assessment. We should consider these results as reassuring; exposure to mainly cannabidiol for up to 16 weeks is safe when quality of life and adaptive behaviour are considered.

Effect of cannabis use in pregnancy

Several large epidemiological studies have reported in detail on the effect of cannabis use during pregnancy. These studies can actually be considered as the ultimate model to study the potential harmful effects on the developing brain. Calvigioni et al. summarized the main results in a review paper in 2014. Data were gathered from three large epidemiological long-term studies: Generation R study (the Netherlands), the Ottawa Prenatal Prospective OPPS study (Ottawa Canada), and the Maternal Health Practices and Child Development MHPCD study (Calvigioni et al., 2014). Although there are many possible methodological shortcomings (such as cumulative dosage, timing of use in pregnancy, and cannabis use before pregnancy), these large studies identify some common short and long-term effects of prenatal cannabis use. Prenatally, there is consistently restricted foetal growth with reduced head circumference. After birth, decreased birth weight and microcephaly are common findings. Some infants show increased startles and tremors with reduced habituation to light. At infant and toddler age, slower psychomotor development can be seen, with subsequent school problems. In particular, impaired memory function, impaired abstract and visual reasoning, or visuospatial functioning are key problem areas. At the behavioural level, more externalising behaviour (hyperactivity and aggressiveness) can be seen. In young adulthood, there is still a possible negative effect on visual spatial memory functioning.

Many of these clinical data have also been confirmed in animal models. In one paper (Tortoriello et al., 2014), reduced synaptic plasticity was observed, which is in line with the hypothesis of exogenous THC effects on presynaptic CB1 receptors (*see above*).

Gunn et al. published a meta-analysis on the effect of prenatal cannabis exposure and included 24 systematic reviews (Gunn et al., 2015). The authors confirmed that infants exposed to *in utero* cannabis were more likely to have decreased birth weight and were more likely to need admission to neonatal intensive care. However, in most studies, it was also recognized that many cannabis users are "polysubstance users"; they are also tobacco and/or alcohol users and the direct unique effects of cannabis were difficult to assess.

More direct evidence is available from neonatal and infant imaging studies. In a recent imaging study, resting state functional brain connectivity was examined in 2-6-week-old babies, after exposure to prenatal drugs, including cannabis (Grewen et al., 2015). In this study, two study groups were defined in order to better delineate the effect of multiple drug use (nicotine, alcohol, SSRI and opiates); one study group with cannabis products (marijuana MJ+) and another group without (MJ-). There was also a control group without any drug exposure in pregnancy. Mainly connections between brain regions known to contain CBD1 receptors were studied. Prenatal drug exposure had a substantial influence on functional connectivity in these infants; marijuana-specific hypo-active connections were observed in insula and striatal connections with the cerebellum: the anterior insula-cerebellum, right caudate-cerebellum, right caudate-right fusiform gyrus/inferior occipital and left caudate-cerebellum. The authors hypothesized that these significant connectivity changes can have an effect on motivation, decision making, and integration of interoceptive signals in later life. However, it remains to be seen whether these connectivity changes at this young age indeed correlate with later cognitive or emotional problems.

Bolhuis et al. (2018) investigated (as part of the generation R study; *see above*) the effects of parental prenatal cannabis exposure on later postnatal 'psychotic-like' experiences.

In this large prospective study (n=3,692), not only the effect of maternal use but also the use of paternal exposure was studied. Not completely surprising, both maternal and paternal cannabis use was associated with psychotic-like experiences at the age of 10 years in the offspring. The authors concluded that both genetic vulnerabilities as well as shared familial mechanisms should be considered when discussing the causal relationship between prenatal cannabis use and postnatal possible psychiatric problems. In their statistical modelling, maternal and paternal age, education level, maternal psychopathology score, and associated alcohol drinking during pregnancy were taken into account as co-variables, but not for later psychotic events. In a similar paper (El Marroun et al., 2019), using the same large generation R cohort, it was also shown that externalisation problems (aggressiveness), in particular, were associated with parental prenatal cannabis exposure, rather than internalising problems such as depression and anxiety.

These large epidemiological studies on prenatal exposure to cannabis show an effect on important developmental functions, and there seems to be more of a pattern with externalizing problems rather than internalising behavioural problems. Long-lasting effects on more subtle higher cognitive functions, such as visuospatial memory, were also noted in several studies.

■ Recreational use in adolescents

One can also look at the effect of recreational cannabis use on the developing brain in adolescents. At this stage in brain development, some specific and especially (pre) frontal functions are still maturing, and repeated use of cannabis might impair these functions. According to many surveys, there is an increased use of cannabis even in young adolescents. Based on an official survey in the US (Miech et al., 2018), it was shown that the lifetime prevalence of cannabis use in 8th graders (14 years old) was between 12.1 and 14.8% (95% confidence limits). This increases up to about 45% (42.8-47.3%) in 12th grade students. Cannabis is now the second most common illicit drug in the US in 12th graders, and about 50% of cannabis users at this age report cannabis use within the last 30 days.

In a review paper on the effects of adolescent cannabis use, based on male and female animal models (Rubino and Parolaro, 2016), it was confirmed that adolescent use dysregulates maturation of the endocannabinoid system which further induces changes in neuronal pruning as well as GABA and glutamate regulation. Many adolescent animal studies show subsequent diminished adapted social behaviour. As expected, these effects depend on dosages of THC and/or other cannabinoids. In a clinical study on connectivity changes in adolescents and young adults using cannabis, increased orbitofrontal connectivity was seen in heavy cannabis smokers, compared to healthy controls (Lopez-Larson et al., 2015). This connectivity change was dose related and increased with lifetime use of cannabis and earlier initiation of cannabis use. The clinical correlate was increased motor impulsivity and suboptimal decision making, again pointing to this possible externalizing problem seen with cannabis use. Another study reported on IQ changes in adults using recreational cannabis and compared two groups: one group with cannabis addiction already before the age of 18 years and one group with cannabis addiction after the age of 18 years (Meier et al., 2012). Participants were part of the Dunedin Study, a prospective study of 1,037 subjects born in 1972/1973 and followed for 38 years. It was clear that adolescent onset of cannabis use was associated with decreased full-scale IQ and this decrease again was dose dependent.

This difference in IQ was less obvious (and not significant) when cannabis use was started at adult ages. The effect size remained after controlling for educational level and other addictions. Overall, this study also showed that baseline IQ was lower in frequent than in infrequent cannabis users. Importantly, cessation of cannabis use in adult age did not fully restore the neuropsychological deficits seen when cannabis was started at adolescent age. The authors conclude that early initiation of cannabis use has a lasting neurotoxic effect on the brain.

Conclusion

So far, there is no direct evidence that the medical use of cannabis derivates for childhood epilepsy is harmful for the developing brain. The short-term controlled trials do not show any major problems, but long-term data in children with epilepsy being treated with cannabis products are needed to confirm this. However, indirect evidence points to a cumulative negative effect on brain development with especially subtle cognitive and behavioural problems. This indirect evidence mainly comes from prenatal and adolescent exposure studies. Here, there are many confounding factors such as cumulative dosage, timing of exposure, and concentration of THC or other cannabinoids.

Epilepsy and cannabidiol: a guide to treatment

**Alexis Arzimanoglou, Ulrich Brandl, J. Helen Cross,
Antonio Gil-Nagel, Lieven Lagae, Cecilie Johannessen Landmark,
Nicola Specchio, Rima Nabbout, Elizabeth A. Thiele,
Oliver Gubbay on behalf of The Cannabinoids International
Experts Panel (*)**

The therapeutic potential of cannabis-related products has been suggested for many years (Perucca, 2017), and interest in the subject in recent decades has fluctuated in parallel with perceptions of cannabis and changes in legislation. With the realisation that (-)-trans-Δ-9-tetrahydrocannabinol (THC) is a component with prominent psychoactive properties, attention shifted to the potential therapeutic value of cannabidiol (CBD). In recent decades, interest in the therapeutic value of CBD-containing products, as anti-inflammatory, anti-emetic, anti-psychotic, and anti-epileptic treatments, has emerged for a wide range of conditions. However, the supporting data is principally based on anecdotal or *in vitro* experiments with supraphysiological concentrations. In addition, other compounds that may be present in artisanal CBD preparations may have independent physiological effects, leading to inevitable confusion regarding the effectiveness and safety of the preparations.

It is only within the last two years that Class I evidence has become available for a pure form of CBD, based on placebo-controlled RCTs. In the light of this recent evidence, this review aims to provide information on the current status of what is known about CBD as a therapeutic option for epilepsy, which will likely be of value to neurologists and epileptologists. This paper contributes to the following competencies of the ILAE curriculum (Blümcke *et al.*, 2019): *"Demonstrate up-to-date knowledge about the range of pharmacological treatments for epilepsy; Recommend appropriate therapy based on epilepsy presentation; Demonstrate up-to-date knowledge about special aspects of pharmacological treatment"*.

(*) Stéphane Auvin (France), Mar Carreno (Spain), Richard Chin (UK), Roberta Cilio (Belgium), Vincenzo Di Marzo (Italy), Maria Del Carmen Fons (Spain), Elaine Hughes (USA), Floor Janssen (The Netherlands), Reetta Kalvilainen (Finland), Tally Lerman-Sagie (Israel), Maria Mazurkiewicz-Bełdzińska (Poland), Nicola Pietrafusa (Italy), Georgia Ramantani (Switzerland), Sylvain Rheims (France), Rocio Sánchez-Carpintero (Spain), Pasquale Striano (Italy), Ben Whalley (UK).

Legislation

Laws regarding the use of raw herbal cannabis, cannabis extracts and cannabinoid-based medicines differ between countries (Abuhasira et al., 2018; Specchio et al., 2020). Recreational use of cannabis has been legalised in Canada and Uruguay, as well as 11 states and the District of Columbia in the US. More restricted recreational use has been adopted in Georgia, South Africa, Spain, and The Netherlands. The use of herbal cannabis for medicinal purposes is now authorised in a number of countries, including Argentina, Australia, Canada, Chile, Colombia, Croatia, Ecuador, Cyprus, Germany, Greece, Israel, Italy, Jamaica, Lithuania, Luxembourg, North Macedonia, Norway, the Netherlands, New Zealand, Peru, Poland, Switzerland, and Thailand, as well as a number of states in the US.

Cannabis and cannabis extracts have not been approved by the FDA or the European Medicines Agency (EMA), although cannabinoid-based products have been approved by the FDA as well as by 23 European countries and Canada. In some cases, authorisation is specific to certain indications, while in others the choice of indication may be dictated by the physician (Abuhasira et al., 2018).

In the European Union, CBD, in contrast to THC, is not a controlled substance and according to EU law, CBD products must not contain more than 0.2% THC. Several companies within the EU produce and distribute CBD-based products obtained from inflorescences of industrial hemp varieties. No analytical controls are mandatory and no legal protection or guarantees regarding the composition and quality is required. An obligatory testing and basic regulatory framework to determine the indication area, daily dosage, route of administration, maximum recommended daily dose, packaging, shelf life, and stability is also not required. Much of the ongoing confusion results from whether such products should be regulated as a food, a supplement, or medicine.

It is beyond the scope of this review to provide details for individual countries. However, physicians considering prescribing cannabis related products should be fully aware of the relevant legislation in relation to the heath care service for their specific geographical location. Since the situation can be complex, provision and use of guidelines from recognised national professional associations and or governmental bodies can be extremely helpful. For example, in the UK, such guidelines have been provided by the British Paediatric Neurology Association (BPNA, 2018) and the National Institute for Health and Care Excellence (NICE, 2019). In both, to prescribe a cannabis related product for medicinal use for epilepsy, the prescriber must be on the Specialist Register (Reference: Section 34D of the Medical Act 1983) and the prescription should be made by a consultant paediatric neurologist. Within the UK, responsibility for the prescribing and potential adverse effects of a cannabis related product remain with the prescribing clinician. Thus, clinicians are advised to be aware of the General Medical Council (GMC) guidance on prescribing unlicensed medication (GMC, 2019), and to investigate whether medical protection insurance and hospital indemnity will cover them for prescription of unlicensed cannabis related products. Should a doctor feel under pressure to prescribe a medication that they believe is not in the patient's interests, then paragraph 5d of the GMC guidance "Consent: patients and doctors making decisions together" is relevant (GMC, 2008). It states: "If the patient asks for a treatment that the doctor considers would not be of overall benefit to them, the doctor should discuss the issues with the patient and explore the reasons for their request. If, after discussion, the doctor still considers that the treatment would not be of overall benefit to the patient, they do not have to provide the treatment. But they should explain their reasons to the patient, and explain any other options that are available, including the option to seek a second opinion".

Artisanal products advertised with CBD content

The known physiologically active components of cannabis include cannabinoids, terpenoids, and flavonoids. Plant or phyto cannabinoids are unique to the cannabis plant. Over a hundred different cannabinoid compounds have been isolated from the cannabis plant, for which various chemovars exist (*Cannabis indica, ruderalis*, and particularly *sativa* being the most common). Of these compounds, only 16 exist in meaningful concentrations; these include THC, CBD, cannabichromene (CBC), and cannabigerol (CBG) (as both acid and varin forms). The majority of animal and *in vitro* studies have focussed on THC and CBD, and whereas the effect of THC is less clear and appears to exhibit both proconvulsant and anticonvulsant properties under different conditions, CBD demonstrates clear anti-convulsant properties, making it a focus as a potential treatment for epilepsy.

An abundance of CBD-related products is currently commercially available, ranging extensively in purity, content of effective compounds and price. The global market for these products is considerable and according to the Centre for Medicinal Cannabis (2019) in the UK, at the current rate, the market will be worth one billion pounds/year in 2025.

Importantly, the content of CBD-related products is dependent on the type of cannabis plant as well as the different parts of the plant and growing conditions. Hemp and marijuana may be considered as different varieties of the same cannabis plant; whereas hemp is low in all cannabinoids including THC (≤ 0.3 %), marijuana has a higher THC content (>0.3%).

Hemp seed oils (from seeds) contain minimal cannabinoids (*i.e.* THC); this depends principally on the extent of washing prior to subsequent processing, as cannabinoids in the flowers and leaves appear to transfer to the outer coating or husk of the seed during harvesting and preparation. Cannabis oils (from flowers and leaves of marijuana) contain variable levels of CBD and THC, depending on the chemovars. CBD-enriched oils (from flowers and leaves of hemp) contain high levels of CBD and some THC. The maximum ratio of CBD to THC that can be achieved without subsequent purification, irrespective of the chemovar, is 20:1, however, it should be noted that THC is significantly more potent (50-100-fold) than CBD. Moreover, for CBD-enriched oils advertised as "high CBD/low THC" content, in order to obtain CBD at similar doses to those used in randomised controlled trials (see below), the meaningful amount of THC may be higher than expected. For a child of 18 kg taking 300 mg CBD/day, this equates to 15 mg THC/day, based on a 20:1 CBD:THC ratio in preparations, which is similar to the maximum daily dosage of marinol or dronabinol, a synthetic Δ-9-THC (prescribed for chemotherapy-induced nausea and vomiting as well as weight loss in cancer or AIDS/HIV patients).

Galenic products are available in the form of cannabis decoction filter bags and cannabis extracts as oils, creams, and supplement capsules. Supplements appear to be the most common form, often referred to as "CBD dietary supplements" or "CBD-enriched oils", obtained from extraction of different *Cannabis sativa L.* chemovars with high CBD content. Of the CBD-enriched oils, there are six main varieties available on the market in Europe: Bedrocan, Bedrobinol, Bediol, Bedica, Bedrolite and Bedropuur (*table 1*).

It is important to emphasise that these products demonstrate significant variation with regards to content, which is dependent not only on the initial source of the plant (*e.g.* the use of fertilisers and pesticides) but also the method by which they are prepared (Carcieri *et al.*, 2018; Pegoraro *et al.*, 2019; Bettiol *et al.*, 2019). There are a number of different methods to prepare such oils, the most common being "supercritical CO_2 extraction". This leads to an extract rich in lipophilic cannabis components plus waxes, however,

Table 1. THC and CBD content of CBD-enriched oils and purified CBD preparations

	Product	THC content	CBD content
CBD-enriched oils	Bedrocan	22%	<1%
	Bedrobinol	13.5%	<1%
	Bediol	6.5%	8%
	Bedica	14%	<1%
	Bedrolite	0.4%	9%
	Bedropuur		<1%
	FM1		
	FM2		
	Pedanios 22/1	22%	<1
	Pedanios 8	8%	8
	Pedanois 1/8	<1%	8
	CBD Crystals 99 %		99%
GW Pharmaceuticals plc	Sativex (GW)	51%	49%
	Epidiolex (GW)		>98%

different biologically active compounds can be isolated during subsequent procedures, including omega-3 fatty acids, vitamins, terpenes, flavonoids, and other phytocannabinoids such as CBC, CBG, cannabidivarin (CBDV), and cannabinol (CBN) as a degradant (according to how the fresh the materials is) (Calvi et al., 2018). Terpenes represent the largest group (with more than 100 different molecules) of cannabis phytochemicals; these can easily cross cell membranes and the blood-brain barrier. Moreover, a synergistic effect between cannabinoids and terpenes has been hypothesised, but not proven (Russo, 2011; Aizpurua-Olaizola et al., 2016; Santiago et al., 2019).

It is also worth mentioning that an adequate dose of CBD based on commercially available CBD-enriched oils (up to 10-20 mg/kg/day), similar to doses used in randomised controlled trials (*see below*), comes at considerable financial cost to the family; in excess of 500 euros per month.

Product labelling

When it comes to CBD-enriched oils, there are major concerns regarding THC, CBD and terpene concentration, as well as appropriate preparation methods and storage conditions. These may vary significantly (Carcieri et al., 2018; Pavlovic et al., 2018), leading to insufficient quality control. Moreover, laboratory analyses have shown that the cannabinoid content is often not reflected on the marketing label (Vandrey et al., 2015).

Based on a report by the Centre for Medicinal Cannabis (2019) in the UK, there is an urgent need for a move towards accurate labelling regarding CBD content, as many products are sold with quantities of CBD which are well below those used in clinical trials. In the study by Bonn-Miller et al. (2017), the label accuracy of 84 products was analysed. Overall, CBD concentration ranged from 0.10 to 655.27 mg/mL (median: 9.45 mg/mL; median labelled concentration: 15.00 mg/mL). Of the products tested, 42.85% (n=36) products were under-labelled, 26.19% (n=22) were over-labelled, and 30.95% (n=26) were accurately labelled. The level of CBD in the over-labelled products in the study is similar in magnitude to levels that triggered a warning from the US Food and Drug Administration (FDA) to 14 businesses in 2015-2016, indicating that there is a continued need for federal and state regulatory agencies to take steps to ensure accurate labelling of these consumer products.

Under-labelling is of less concern, as CBD itself does not appear to be susceptible to abuse and there have been no reported serious adverse effects (AEs) at high doses, however, the THC content observed may be sufficient to produce intoxication or impairment, especially among children. Clear labelling regarding the exact concentration of CBD is not yet mandatory, and there is clearly a need to introduce stricter legislation regarding accurate content labelling.

Effectiveness as a treatment for epilepsy

Anecdotal reports have fuelled public interest and, understandably, have inspired families to seek CBD-related products for the treatment of drug-resistant epilepsy (Filloux, 2015). The most well-known report is that of Charlotte, a five-year-old girl in the US who was diagnosed in 2013 with *SCN1A*-confirmed Dravet syndrome, with up to 50 generalised tonic-clonic seizures per day. Following three months of treatment with high-CBD-strain cannabis extract (later marketed as "Charlotte's Web"), her seizures were reported to have reduced by more than 90% (Maa and Figi, 2014). Other anecdotal reports suggesting that CBD may improve seizure control as well as alertness, mood and sleep have also been documented (Porter and Jacobson, 2013; Hussain *et al.*, 2015; Schonhofen *et al.*, 2018).

A number of studies have investigated the effect of oral cannabis extracts on intractable epilepsy, based on parental reporting. These include the study by Press *et al.* (2015) of 75 patients (23% with Dravet syndrome and 89% with Lennox-Gastaut syndrome) in the US and Tzadok *et al.* (2016) of 74 patients in Israel over an average of six months; 50% seizure reduction was reported in 33%, and 50-75% seizure reduction in 34% in the two studies, respectively. In a retrospective study by Porcari *et al.* (2018) of 108 children with epilepsy in the US, the addition of CBD oil over an average of six months resulted in >50% seizure reduction in 29% patients, with 10% becoming seizure-free.

Based on a meta-analysis (n=670), Pamplona *et al.* (2018) provide evidence in support of the therapeutic value of high-content CBD treatments (CBD-rich cannabis extract or purified CBD). The results indicated a favourable effect for both patients with CBD-rich extracts (6.1 mg/kg/day CBD) and purified CBD (27.1 mg/kg/day), which was in fact more pronounced in patients taking the CBD-rich extracts. This may provide evidence in favour of the inclusion of other components within CBD-rich extracts offering beneficial entourage effects.

Overall, the studies on CBD-enriched oils indicate a 50% reduction in seizures in roughly 30-40% patients. However, it should be emphasised that these are uncontrolled studies with heterogeneous CBD preparations, the CBD content of which varied significantly (estimated at <0.02-50 mg/kg/day). In the study of Press *et al.* (2015), the effect of cannabis extracts was investigated in a cohort of paediatric patients with epilepsy in a single tertiary epilepsy centre in Colorado, where the law on cannabis-related products is more relaxed.

Interestingly, the overall responder rate (47%) for patients who had moved to Colorado for treatment was greater than that (22%) of those who were already living in Colorado, indicating a possible positive reporting bias and the need for appropriately controlled studies.

Adverse events

The studies described above reported AEs in 40-50% patients, including increased seizure frequency, gastrointestinal disturbances/diarrhoea, appetite alteration, weight changes, nausea, liver dysfunction, pancreatitis and, particularly, somnolence and fatigue. More serious effects included developmental regression, abnormal movements and status epilepticus.

More long-term effects regarding cannabis-derived products have generally been gathered based on indirect evidence, however, no hard conclusions can be drawn, mainly due to methodological limitations (dosage of THC and other cannabis-derived products, duration of exposure, concordant addiction to other drugs, genetic factors, psychiatric comorbidity, *etc.*). Long-term data from studies on prenatal and adolescent exposure to cannabis products indicate, however, a possible negative and lasting effect on cognitive and, particularly, behavioural functions (Lagae, 2020). Moreover, the externalisation of behavioural problems and a decrease in IQ have been reported as a result of chronic cannabis use. Clearly, long-term studies using large childhood epilepsy cohorts are needed on the chronic use of CBD and cannabis-related products.

■ Purified CBD (Epidiolex/Epidyolex®)

A purified preparation of CBD is available from GW Pharmaceuticals plc, under the name of Epidiolex/Epidyolex® (>98% CBD). Interest has so far largely focussed on Epidiolex as an add-on drug for cases of epilepsy. Another product, Sativex® (also known as Nabiximol) (51% THC, 49% CBD), made by the same company as a refined extract, has been approved for cases of neuropathic pain, spasticity, overactive bladder and other symptoms of multiple sclerosis in some countries.

Purified CBD has been shown to demonstrate positive effects against a wide spectrum of seizures and epilepsy based on animal models (Rosenburg *et al.*, 2017a). While the precise mechanism of action of CBD in the control of epileptic seizures in humans remains unknown, recent evidence suggests a role in modulating intracellular Ca^{2+} (including effects on neuronal Ca^{2+} mobilisation via GPR55 and TRPV1) and modulating adenosine-mediated signalling (Gray and Whalley, 2020).

In 2017 and 2018, the first randomised controlled trials for pharmaceutically prepared Epidiolex were published for Dravet syndrome and Lennox-Gastaut syndrome, respectively (Devinsky *et al.*, 2017; Thiele *et al.*, 2018), and in June 2018, the FDA approved CBD as an add-on antiepileptic drug for patients with Lennox-Gastaut syndrome or Dravet syndrome over the age of two. Epidiolex was also later approved by the EMA in September 2019 for patients over two years of age with Dravet syndrome and Lennox-Gastaut syndrome, in conjunction with clobazam. However, accessibility to Epidiolex outside of Europe and the US remains variable (*e.g.* only patients involved in RCTs may be eligible), due to a lack of approval and legal reform by central agencies. While such reform is clearly welcomed, it cannot come fast enough for those who may benefit.

Pharmacology and drug interactions

As a therapeutic drug, the pharmacokinetic profile of CBD exhibits low bioavailability, significant protein binding (99% protein binding capability), and interactions with various metabolic pathways in the liver, including CYPs that are susceptible to pharmacogenetic variability and drug interactions. However, as CBD interacts with many enzymes, it is cleared quickly and is therefore less susceptible to modulation by drugs that affect metabolising enzymes. Moreover, the pharmacokinetic profile of CBD seems relatively unaffected by inhibitors and inducers or genetic background. The bioavailability of oral oil formulations is limited (<6%) due to extensive first pass metabolism in the liver (Bialer et al., 2017, 2018).

CBD may exhibit numerous interactions with AEDs (Johannessen Landmark and Patsalos, 2010; Johannessen and Johannessen Landmark, 2010; Johannessen Landmark et al., 2012, 2016; Patsalos, 2013a, 2013b) including both potent enzyme inducers (such as carbamazepine and phenytoin) and inhibitors (such as stiripentol, felbamate and valproate) (table 2), however, the clinical significance of these interactions may not be meaningful. The most obvious and clinically significant interaction between CBD and other concomitantly used drugs, based on clinical trials, is that with clobazam. CBD, via enzyme inhibition (CYP2C19), may lead to an increase (up to five-fold) in its less potent metabolite, N-desmethylclobazam (Geffrey et al., 2015; Devinsky et al., 2018a), leading to toxicity (principally manifesting as sedation [Gaston et al., 2017]), which may occur at even low levels (1 mg/kg/day) (unpublished observations; Johannessen Landmark). In addition, concurrent clobazam may lead to increased 7-hydroxy-cannabidiol (an active metabolite of CBD) (Morrison et al., 2019), which arguably may lead to better seizure control by boosting the effect of CBD, however, studies with and without clobazam are needed to confirm this. Other AEDs with a similarly increased effect, concomitant with CBD, may include topiramate, rufinamide, zonisamide and eslicarbazepine (Gaston et al., 2017; Franco and Perucca, 2019). There are therefore still a number of unanswered questions regarding the pharmacology of CBD (Johannessen Landmark and Brandl, 2020; Brodie and Ben-Menachem, 2018).

The clinical impact of such interactions in the individual patient is difficult to predict. Patients should be systematically questioned about efficacy, tolerability and adherence, and serum concentrations should be measured if possible and dosages adjusted accordingly to optimise each patient's treatment.

Table 2. Possible AED/CBD interactions

Enzyme inducer (↓)	Enzyme inhibitor (↑)	CBD as an enzyme inhibitor (↑)
Carbamazepine	Valproate*	Clobazam**
Phenytoin	Stiripentol	Topiramate
	Felbamate	Rufinamide
		Zonisamide
		Eslicarbazepine
		Perampanel
		Lamotrigine?

* Associated with a significant risk of elevated transaminases.
** Associated with a significant risk of elevated N-desmethylclobazam, which may cause e.g. sedation.

Efficacy as a treatment for epilepsy

The first trials for purified CBD (Epidiolex) were launched as an expanded access programme in 2014 for patients with significant medically refractory epilepsy in the form of an open-label, non-controlled trial for compassionate use (Devinsky et al., 2016). Patients (n=214) with intractable seizures (at least four weekly) were monitored over a 12-week period (relative to a four-week baseline) with initial CBD doses of 2.5-5 mg/kg/day, increasing weekly to 25 or 50 mg/kg/day. Overall, a 36.5% median reduction of motor seizures was reported (49.8% for Dravet syndrome patients), and five patients were free of all motor seizures (of the patients with motor and atonic seizures, 39% and 56% showed a >50% reduction of seizures, respectively). This programme was continued and interim data on >600 patients over a 96-week period were published in 2018 by Szaflarski et al., revealing a reduction of median monthly convulsive seizures by 51% (52% with ≥50% seizure reduction) and total seizures by 48% at 12 weeks, with similar results over the 96-week period.

With these very encouraging results, shortly after the initial launch of this programme, controlled trials for Epidiolex were established for Dravet syndrome (Devinsky et al., 2017) and Lennox-Gastaut syndrome (Thiele et al., 2018; Devinsky et al., 2018b). For further details regarding these trials, refer to Nabbout and Thiele (2020).

Lennox Gastaut syndrome

In the two Lennox-Gastaut syndrome double-blind placebo-controlled trials, patients (n=171 and 225) were administered CBD at 20 mg/kg/day (GWPCARE4; Thiele et al., 2018) or 10 or 20 mg/kg/day (GWPCARE3; Devinsky et al., 2018b) over a 14-week treatment period (including a titration phase of two weeks starting with a dose of 2.5 mg/kg/day, titrated to 10 or 20 mg/kg/day), and data were compared relative to a four-week baseline observation period. CBD in an oral solution or placebo was administered as add-on to current AEDs. For CBD at 20 mg/kg/day, the median percentage reduction in total seizure frequency was 41% (vs 13.7% placebo) and 38.4% (vs 18.5% placebo), and monthly median decrease in drop seizures was reported to be 44% (vs 22% placebo) and 42% (vs 17% placebo) in the two trials, respectively. At 10 mg/kg/day, the median percentage reduction in total seizure frequency was similar at 36.4% (vs 18.5% placebo), and monthly median decrease in drop seizures was 37% (vs 17% placebo).

Lennox-Gastaut syndrome patients who enrolled in these RCTs were also invited to enter an open-label study (GWPCARE5; Thiele et al., 2019a). The interim data after 48 weeks of treatment revealed a 48-60% median decrease in drop seizure frequency and a 48-57% median decrease in monthly total seizure frequency relative to baseline (figure 1).

Based on the patient or caregiver Clinical Global Impression (CGI) scale, overall improvements were reported in patients of each trial: 58% patients (compared to 34% in the placebo group) in the study of Thiele et al. (2018), 57% and 66% in the 20 mg/kg/day and 10 mg/kg/day group, respectively (compared to 44% in the placebo group) in the study of Devinsky et al. (2018b), and 88% at 24 weeks (also similar at 38 and 48 weeks) in the open-label study of Thiele et al. (2019a).

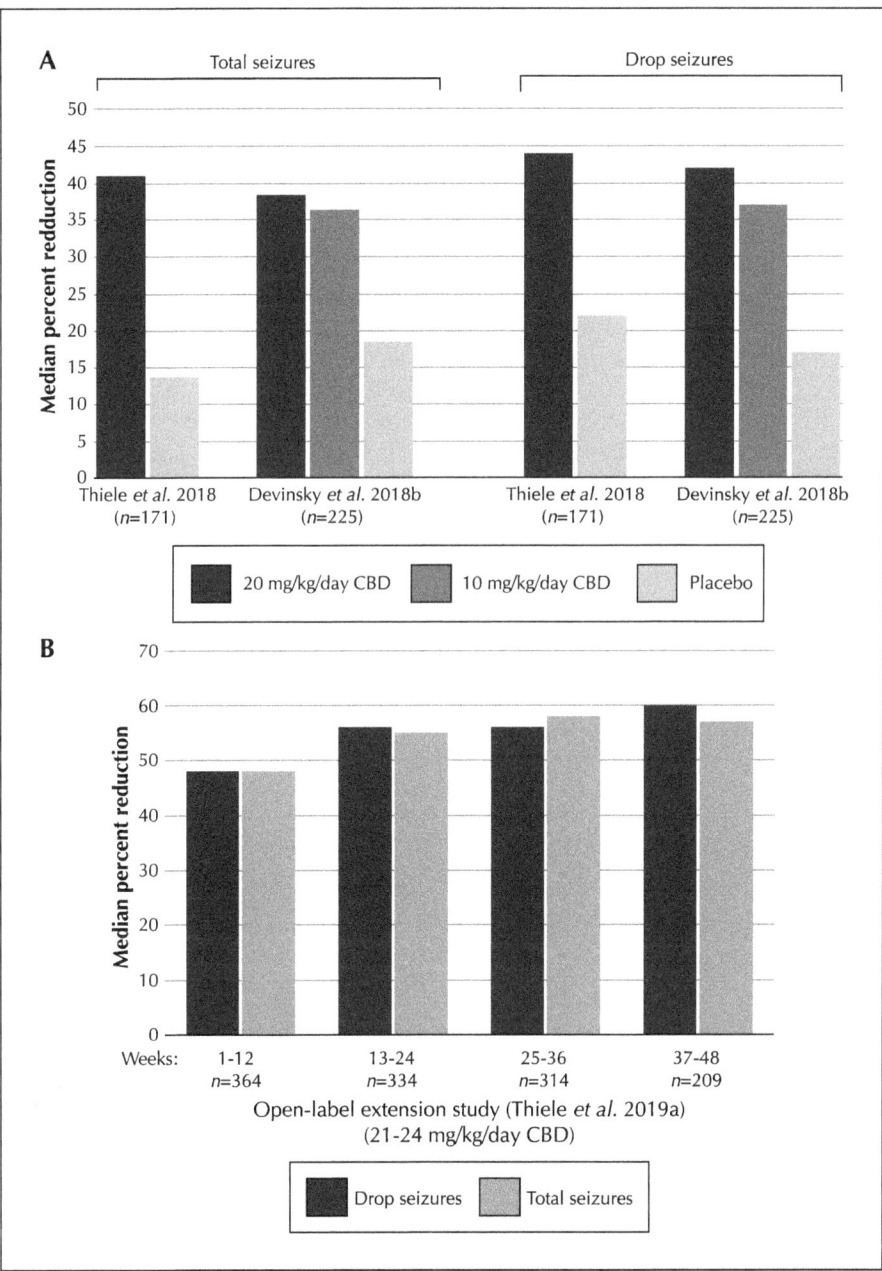

Figure 1/ Median percent reduction of Lennox-Gastaut syndrome total seizures and monthly drop seizures based on the two controlled trials (Thiele et al., 2018; Devinsky et al., 2018b) (A), and the open-label extension study (Thiele et al., 2019a) (B).

Dravet syndrome

For Dravet syndrome, two trials involved an initial double-blind placebo-controlled trial (n=120) (GWPCARE1B; Devinsky et al., 2017) and a later open-label extension programme (GWPCARE5; Devinsky et al., 2019). An additional trial has also recently been completed (GWPCARE2; Miller et al., 2019). For the former, similar to the Lennox-Gastaut syndrome trials, patients were administered 20 mg/kg/day CBD over a 14-week treatment period, and data were compared relative to a four-week baseline period. For the open-label extension programme, a subset of these patients together with participants from the recently completed GWPCARE2 trial were enlisted (n=189) and followed over 48 weeks. For the controlled trial, during the treatment period, the median percent reduction of convulsive seizures and total seizures was 39% and 29% in the CBD arm relative to 13% and 9% in the placebo arm, respectively. The difference in median percent reduction in non-convulsive seizures was not significant. During the open-label extension programme, the median percent reduction of total seizures continued at between 39% and 51% over a 48-week period (*figure 2*).

As part of the expanded access programme mentioned above, the long-term effect of add-on CBD at up to 25-50 mg/kg/day over a period of 144 weeks was reported for Dravet syndrome and Lennox-Gastaut syndrome patients (Laux et al., 2019). Monthly major motor seizures were reduced by 50% and total seizures by 44%, with consistent reductions in both seizure types across the treatment period, thus supporting CBD as a long-term treatment option. Based on the patient or caregiver CGI scale, overall improvements were reported for both trials: 62% patients (compared to 34% in the placebo arm) in the study of Devinsky et al. (2017), and 85% at 48 weeks in the open-label study of Devinsky et al. (2019).

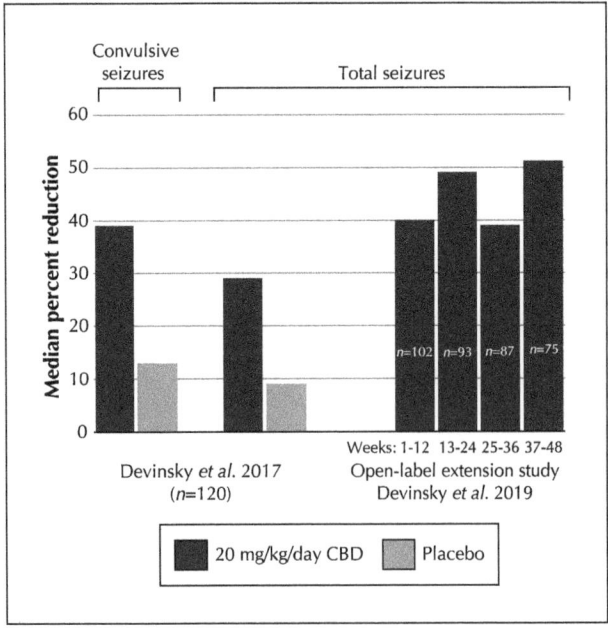

Figure 2/ Median percent reduction of Dravet syndrome total seizures and convulsive seizures based on the controlled trial of Devinsky et al. (2017) and the open-label extension programme of Devinsky et al. (2019).

Tuberous sclerosis complex

A clinical trial (GWPCARE6) for Epidiolex as add-on treatment in patients with tuberous sclerosis complex (TSC) was completed earlier this year and has also revealed promising results (Thiele et al., 2019b). Patients were randomised into two groups with Epidiolex (25 or 50 mg/kg/day) or placebo. Of the 201 patients who completed the study, total seizure frequency was decreased by 48% ($p=0.0013$), 48% ($p=0.0018$) and 27%, and 50% seizure reduction in 36% ($p=0.0692$), 40% ($p=0.0245$), and 22% in the 20 mg/kg/day, 50 mg/kg/day and placebo groups, respectively. An overall improvement, based on the caregiver CGI scale, was reported for 69% ($p=0.0074$), 62% ($p=0.580$) and 40% in the three groups, respectively. In conclusion, Epidiolex significantly reduced seizures in TSC patients. The therapeutic effect of the lower 25 mg/kg/day concentration was similar to that of the higher 50 mg/kg/day dose, and since the latter was associated with more AEs (see below), the 25 mg/kg/day dose would therefore be indicated for these patients.

Other syndromes

Based on an open-label trial for compassionate use, CBD was tested as a treatment for CDKL5 deficiency disorder and Aicardi, Doose, and Dup15q syndromes over a 12-week period ($n=55$) (Devinsky et al., 2018c). The mean decrease in convulsive seizure frequency was 51.4% ($n=35$). Studies are underway to evaluate CBD efficacy for a broader range of epilepsy syndromes and more than 20 trials are currently listed at ClinicalTrials.gov.

Overall, evidence from open-label studies suggests a favourable effect of CBD as an add-on treatment for a number of severe epileptic conditions and the controlled trials for Lennox-Gastaut syndrome, Dravet syndrome and TSC provide a clearer picture of the positive effect of CBD, in some cases even correlating with seizure freedom. A general positive trend for quality of life (particularly in Lennox-Gastaut syndrome patients), sleep behaviour (particularly in Dravet syndrome patients) and adaptive behaviour was reported. There were also particular improvements in the socialisation domain and communication domain for Dravet syndrome and Lennox-Gastaut syndrome patients, respectively. In the prospective, open-label clinical study by Rosenberg et al. (2017b), in which caregiver-reported quality of life ($n=48$) was evaluated for a subset of patients treated with CBD for 12 weeks, improvements (in energy/fatigue, memory, control/helplessness, other cognitive functions, social interactions, behaviour and global QOL) were not related to changes in seizure frequency or AEs, suggesting that CBD may have beneficial effects on patient QOL, distinct from anti-seizure effects, however, this should be confirmed in controlled studies.

Adverse effects

In contrast to artisanal CBD-related products, the AEs associated with purified CBD have been more clearly demonstrated based on the open-label trials and, particularly, the randomised, double-blind placebo-controlled trials (Anciones and Gil-Nagel, 2020).

Based on the collective data from the controlled trials, AEs were frequently reported (86% in CBD groups and 76% in placebo groups), however, the vast majority of AEs were mild and moderate. These included somnolence, decreased appetite, pyrexia and diarrhoea, followed by other less frequent AEs such as vomiting, fatigue and upper respiratory infections (*table 3*). Most AEs appeared within the first two weeks of treatment. Serious AEs were far

Table 3. Adverse events based on randomised, double-blind, placebo-controlled trials (the most frequent adverse events are highlighted in grey)

	Dravet syndrome				Lennox-Gastaut syndrome			
	Devinsky et al., 2017		Devinsky et al., 2018a		Devinsky et al., 2018b		Thiele et al., 2018	
	CBD (n=61)	Placebo (n=59)	CBD (n=27)	Placebo (n=7)	CBD (n=149)	Placebo (n=76)	CBD (n=86)	Placebo (n=85)
[CBD] mg/kg/day	20	-	5, 10 or 20	-	10 or 20	-	20	-
Reported AEs (%)	93	75	74	86	89	72	86	69
Reported serious AEs (n)	10	3	5	1	26	13	20	4
Withdrawn (n)	8	1	2	-	7	1	12	1
Somnolence (n)*a	22	6	5	1	39	4	25	15
Decreased appetite (n)	17	3	5	0	32	6	19	3
Pyrexia (n)*	9	5	6	0	16	12	12	8
Diarrhoea (n)	19	6			19	6	27	10
Elevated transaminases (n)*b	12	1	6	-	14	0	20	1
Vomiting (n)	9	3	3	0	10	9	15	18
Fatigue (n)	12	2	1	2				
Upper respiratory infections (n)	7	5			21	11		
Pharyngitis (n)			3	2	12	5		
Convulsion (n)*	7	3	1	2				
Sedation (n)			4	0				
Ataxia (n)			3	0				
Rash (n)*			2	0				
Non-specified pneumonia (n)			2	0				
Lethargy (n)*	8	3						
Status epilepticus (n)	3	3			11	3	1	1

* Serious adverse events reported in ≤2 patients per RCT.
a Majority of patients were also taking clobazam.
b >79% patients were taking valproate (transaminases were elevated >3 times the upper normal limit).

less common (affecting 19% of CBD groups and 9% of placebo groups). These included, in particular, somnolence, pyrexia, convulsion, rash, lethargy and elevated transaminases (>three times the normal upper limit). The latter occurred in 16% patients in the CBD groups and 1% in the placebo groups. Moreover, in >79-100% of the cases with elevated transaminases, patients were concomitantly taking valproate.

No seizure worsening, suicidal ideation or deaths related to the treatment were reported. It should be emphasised, however, given the novelty of Epidiolex, that long-term AEs are currently unknown.

In the recent TSC trial with the higher dose of 50 mg/kg/day CBD (Thiele et al., 2019b), AEs were common but similarly overall reported as mild and moderate (93%, 100% and 95% in the 25 mg/kg/day; 50 mg/kg/day and placebo groups, respectively). The most common AEs were diarrhoea, decreased appetite, and somnolence, and treatment discontinuation due to AEs occurred in 11%, 14% and 3%, respectively. Elevated liver enzymes were reported in 12% (n=9) and 25% (n=18) in the 25 mg/kg/day and 50 mg/kg/day, respectively (of those, 81% were also taking valproate).

Recommendations for use

CBD is administered orally as an oil solution. In open-label studies, doses mostly up to 25 mg/kg/day were used, and in the controlled studies, higher doses up to 50 mg/kg/day were used. The studies on Lennox-Gastaut syndrome, however, show that a significant proportion of children respond to doses of as little as 10 mg/kg/day. Therefore a "start slow" and "increase on a case-by-case basis" strategy is recommended. A starting dose of 5 mg/kg/day, divided in two doses, would appear to be adequate. This dose should be increased to 10 mg/kg/day after two weeks of treatment. Thereafter, the individual's response should be carefully observed. The required observation time strictly depends on baseline seizure frequency before the administration of CBD. If the drug is well tolerated but not sufficiently effective, the dose should be slowly increased in increments of 5 mg/kg/day, as long as it is tolerated, up to a maximum of 20-25 mg/kg/day (*table 4*).

As mentioned above, special care should be taken if both CBD and clobazam are administered, since the addition of CBD may lead to an increase (up to five-fold) in its less potent metabolite, N-desmethylclobazam. A toxic benzodiazepine level may manifest as fatigue, somnolence, ataxia, a decrease in cognitive function or behavioural changes. Clinically, these are difficult to distinguish from the possible AEs of CBD itself and monitoring of clobazam/N-desmethylclobazam levels is therefore recommended. Baseline therapeutic drug monitoring should be performed before administration of CBD and subsequently after each increase. If a significant increase in benzodiazepine level is observed, the dose of clobazam should be reduced (and then checked), according to an estimate based on linear kinetics. Like CBD, however, stiripentol inhibits the same P450 subtype 2C19 (CYP2C19), and an increase in benzodiazepine level may not, therefore, occur if the patient is already on stiripentol (Devinsky et al., 2018b). It is highly recommended to follow serum concentrations of all drugs when initiating CBD as a basis for appropriate dosage adjustment. This includes psychotropic drugs (mood stabilisers, antidepressants, and antipsychotics) in order to reveal possible pharmacokinetic interactions or reasons for poor clinical effects or observed AEs.

Table 4. Guide to CBD dosing

1	Start low (5 mg/kg/day), increase to 10 mg/kg/day after two weeks
2	Review clinical response and adverse effects at 10 mg/kg/day
3	Remain on this dose if effective, otherwise increase dose in steps of 5 mg/kg/day if CBD is well tolerated
4	Stop at 20-25 mg/kg/day, and withdraw CBD if ineffective

Pharmacogenetic testing for CYP2C19 could be performed if a poor metabolizer genotype is suspected based on unexpectedly high levels of CBD relative to the dose.

Finally, biochemical markers of toxicity should be measured, particularly regarding liver enzymes in conjunction with valproate (Gaston *et al.*, 2017; Devinsky *et al.*, 2018a). In the controlled studies, increased liver enzymes led to withdrawal of CBD if levels were more than three times the upper normal limit in the presence of any symptoms (fever, rash, nausea, abdominal pain or increased bilirubin) or eight times higher in the absence of such symptoms. In rare cases, an increase in enzymes was observed with 20 mg/kg/day CBD without concomitant use of valproate, but not with lower doses of CBD. Overall, the increase in liver enzymes was reversible in about half the cases, without taking any action; in the remaining cases, CBD was withdrawn, leading to normalisation of levels (Devinsky *et al.*, 2018b). A mild increase in enzyme levels may be observed over a few weeks before taking any action, however, as levels become too high, CBD or valproate should be withdrawn or reduced, according to the benefit of each.

■ Conclusions

Given the range of, and easy access to CBD-enriched oils on the market, alongside the fallacious perception that "natural" products may be safer with fewer AEs than conventional AEDs, it is clear to see why such products are popular. However, analytical controls for CBD-enriched products are not mandatory, leaving consumers with no legal protection or guarantees about the composition and quality of the product they are acquiring. Currently, CBD-enriched products are not subject to any obligatory testing or basic regulatory framework to determine the indication area, daily dosage, route of administration, maximum recommended daily dose, packaging, shelf life or stability. The content of these products is therefore highly variable and although components other than CBD are present which may even be beneficial, there is currently no way this can be ascertained or controlled.

In contrast, purified CBD, in the form of Epidiolex/Epidyolex, is a standardised pharmaceutical preparation that is subject to minimal variability. Based on controlled trials, Epidiolex appears to be an effective treatment option for patients with Dravet syndrome, Lennox-Gastaut syndrome and TSC and has a relatively good safety profile, although it should be emphasised that, at least from the controlled trials, CBD does not outperform other drugs and will by no means represent a silver bullet for everyone. It does, however, add to the arsenal of available add-on drugs against these severe forms of epilepsy, in some cases offering substantial benefits.

Given the range of different seizure types associated with Dravet syndrome, Lennox-Gastaut syndrome and TSC, CBD would appear to have a favourable effect on a large spectrum of convulsive (consistent with preclinical data), rather than non-convulsive seizures (Devinsky *et al.*, 2017), namely clonic, myoclonic, myoclonic-astatic, and generalised tonic-clonic seizures. It should be noted, however, that the effect of CBD on specific types of seizures was not described in detail in the controlled trials and further studies will therefore be required to address this. Other forms of intractable epilepsy cases have been investigated in open-label trials (CDKL5 deficiency disorder and Aicardi, Dup15q and Doose syndromes; Devinsky *et al.*, [2018c]), and more than 20 trials are currently listed at ClinicalTrials.gov (including Rett syndrome and other forms of intractable epilepsy). Although these syndromes collectively represent a small fraction of the epilepsy population, clinical trials in the future may lead to CBD or indeed other cannabinoids being indicated more broadly across the spectrum of epilepsy syndromes.

Bibliography

Abuhasira R, Shbiro L, Landschaft Y. Medical use of cannabis and cannabinoids containing products - Regulations in Europe and North America. *Eur J Intern Med* 2018;49:2–6.

Aggarwal SK, Blinderman CD. Cannabis for symptom control #279. *J Palliat Med* 2014;17(5):612–4.

Aizpurua-Olaizola O, Soydaner U, Öztürk E, et al. Evolution of the cannabinoid and terpene content during the growth of cannabis sativa plants from different chemotypes. *J Nat Prod* 2016;79:324–31.

American Psychiatric Association. Diagnostic and Statistical Manual of Mental Disorders. 5th ed. Arlington, VA: American Psychiatric Publishing; 2013.

Ames FR, Cridland S. Anticonvulsant effect of cannabidiol. *S Afr Med J* 1986;69(1):14.

Amorim BO, Hamani C, Ferreira E, et al. Effects of A1 receptor agonist/antagonist on spontaneous seizures in pilocarpine-induced epileptic rats. *Epilepsy Behav* 2016;61:168–73.

Anciones C, Gil-Nagel A. Adverse effects of cannabinoids. *Epileptic Disord* 2020;22(Suppl. 1):S29–32.

Arzimanoglou A, Brandl U, Cross JH, et al. Epilepsy and cannabidiol: a guide to treatment. *Epileptic Disord* 2020;22:1–14.

Atsmon J, Cherniakov I, Izgelov D, et al. PTL401, a new formulation based on pro-nano-dispersion technology, improves oral cannabinoids bioavailability in health volunteers. *J Pharm Sci* 2018;107:1423–9.

Australian Government Department of Health Therapeutic Goods Administration. Books. https://www.tga.gov.au/book/part-final-decisions-matters-referred-expert-advisory-committee-2.

Bakas T, van Nieuwenhuijzen PS, Devenish SO, McGregor IS, Arnold JC, Chebib M. The direct actions of cannabidiol and 2-arachidonoyl glycerol at GABAA receptors. *Pharmacol Res* 2017;119:358–70.

Barnes MP. Sativex: clinical efficacy and tolerability in the treatment of symptoms of multiple sclerosis and neuropathic pain. *Expert Opin Pharmacother* 2006;7(5):607–15.

Beal JE, Olson R, Lefkowitz L, et al. Long-term efficacy and safety of dronabinol for acquired immunodeficiency syndrome-associated anorexia. *J Pain Symptom Manage* 1997;14(1):7–14.

Bestard JA, Toth CC. An open-label comparison of nabilone and gabapentin as adjuvant therapy or monotherapy in the management of neuropathic pain in patients with peripheral neuropathy. *Pain Pract* 2011;11(4):353–68.

Bettiol A, Lombardi N, Crescioli G, et al. Galenic preparations of therapeutic cannabis sativa differ in cannabinoids concentration: a quantitative analysis of variability and possible clinical implications. *Front Pharmacol* 2019;9:1543.

Bialer M, Johannessen SI, Koepp MJ, et al. Progress report on new antiepileptic drugs: a summary of the Fourteenth Eilat Conference on New Antiepileptic Drugs and Devices (EILAT XIV). II. Drugs in more advanced clinical development. *Epilepsia* 2018;59:1842–66.

Bialer M, Johannessen SI, Levy RH, Perucca E, Tomson T, White HS. Progress report on new antiepileptic drugs: A summary of the Thirteenth Eilat Conference on New Antiepileptic Drugs and Devices (EILAT XIII). *Epilepsia* 2017;58(2):181–221.

Bisogno T, Hanus L, De Petrocellis L, et al. Molecular targets for cannabidiol and its synthetic analogues: effect on vanilloid VR1 receptors and on the cellular uptake and enzymatic hydrolysis of anandamide. *Br J Pharmacol* 2001;134(4):845–52.

Blümcke I, Arzimanoglou A, Beniczky S, Wiebe S. Roadmap for a competency-based educational curriculum in epileptology: report of the Epilepsy Education Task Force of the ILAE. *Epileptic Disord* 2019;21:129–40.

Boison D. The biochemistry and epigenetics of epilepsy: focus on adenosine and glycine. *Front Mol Neurosci* 2016;9:26.

Bolhuis K, Kushner SA, Yalniz S, et al. Maternal and paternal cannabis use during pregnancy and the risk of psychotic-like experiences in the offspring. *Schizophr Res* 2018;202:322–7.

Bonn-Miller MO, Loflin MJE, Thomas BF, Marcu JP, Hyke T, Vandrey R. Labeling accuracy of cannabidiol extracts sold online. *JAMA* 2017;318(17):1708–9.

Borgelt LM, Franson KL, Nussbaum AM, Wang GS. The pharmacologic and clinical effects of medical cannabis. *Pharmacotherapy* 2013;33(2):195–209.

Bossong MG, Niesink RJ. Adolescent brain maturation, the endogenous cannabinoid system and the neurobiology of cannabis-induced schizophrenia. *Prog Neurobiol* 2010;92:370–85.

BPNA. *Guidance on the use of cannabis-based products for medicinal use in children and young people with epilepsy.* 2018. https://bpna.org.uk/userfiles/BPNA_CBPM_Guidance_Oct2018.pdf.

Brodie MJ, Ben-Menachem E. Cannabinoides for epilepsy : What do we know and where do we go ? *Epilepsia* 2018;59:291–6.

Brown AJ, Wise A. Identification of modulators of GPR55 activity. 2001. WO2001086305A3.

Burns ML, Baftiu A, Opdahl MS, Johannessen SI, Johannessen Landmark C. Therapeutic drug monitoring of clobazam and its metabolite -impact of age and comedication on pharmacokinetic variability. *Ther Drug Monit* 2016;38:350–7.

Calvi L, Pentimalli D, Panseri S, et al. Comprehensive quality evaluation of medical Cannabis sativa L. inflorescence and macerated oils based on HS-SPME coupled to GC-MS and LC-HRMS (q-exactive orbitrap®) approach. *J Pharm Biomed Anal* 2018;150:208–19.

Calvigioni D, Hurd YL, Harkany T, Keimpema E. Neuronal substrates and functional consequences of prenatal cannabis exposure. *Eur Child Adolesc Psychiatry* 2014;23(10):931–41.

Canada: Government of Canada Justice Laws Website. *Controlled Drugs and Substances Act.* http://laws-lois.justice.gc.ca/eng/acts/c-38.8/FullText.html.

Carcieri C, Tomasello C, Simiele M. Cannabinoids concentration variability in cannabis olive oil galenic preparations. *J Pharm Pharmacol* 2018;70(1):143–9.

Caterina MJ, Schumacher MA, Tominaga M, Rosen TA, Levine JD, Julius D. The capsaicin receptor: a heat-activated ion channel in the pain pathway. *Nature* 1997;389:816–24.

Centre for Medicinal Canabis. *UK CBD Requires Better Regulation and Reform as Industry Moves Towards Billion Pound Sector Status.* 2019. https://www.thecmcuk.org/uk_cbd_requires_better_regulation.

Chiron C, Kassai B, Dulac O, Pons G, Nabbout R. A revisited strategy for antiepileptic drug development in children: designing an initial exploratory step. *CNS Drugs* 2013;27(3):185–95.

Chung JM, Lee KH, Hori Y, Willis WD. Effects of capsaicin applied to a peripheral nerve on the responses of primate spinothalamic tract cells. *Brain Res* 1985;329:27–38.

Cunha JM, Carlini EA, Pereira AE, et al. Chronic administration of cannabidiol to healthy volunteers and epileptic patients. *Pharmacology* 1980;21(3):175–85.

DAC. *Neu in DAC/NRF: Cannabidiol*. 2015 http://dacnrf.pharmazeutische-zeitung.de/index.php ?id=557.

de Leon J, Spina E, Diaz FJ. Clobazam therapeutic drug monitoring: a comprehensive review of the literature with proposals to improve future studies. *Ther Drug Monit* 2013;35:30–47.

De Liso P, Chemaly N, Laschet J, et al. Patients with Dravet syndrome in the era of stiripentol: a French cohort cross-sectional study. *Epilepsy Res* 2016;125:42–6.

De Petrocellis L, Ligresti A, Moriello AS, et al. Effects of cannabinoids and cannabinoid-enriched Cannabis extracts on TRP channels and endocannabinoid metabolic enzymes. *Br J Pharmacol* 2011;163(7):1479–94.

De Petrocellis L, Nabissi M, Santoni G, Ligresti A. Actions and regulation of ionotropic cannabinoid receptors. *Adv Pharmacol* 2017;80:249–89.

Devinsky O, Cilio MR, Cross H, et al. Cannabidiol: pharmacology and potential therapeutic role in epilepsy and other neuropsychiatric disorders. *Epilepsia* 2014;55(6):791–802.

Devinsky O, Cross JH, Laux L, et al. Trial of cannabidiol for drug-resistant seizures in the dravet syndrome. *N Engl J Med* 2017;376(21):2011–20.

Devinsky O, Cross JH, Wright S. Trial of cannabidiol for drug-resistant seizures in the Dravet syndrome. *N Engl J Med* 2017;377(7):699–700.

Devinsky O, Marsh E, Friedman D, et al. Cannabidiol in patients with treatment-resistant epilepsy: an open-label interventional trial. *Lancet Neurol* 2016;15(3):270–8.

Devinsky O, Nabbout R, Miller I, et al. Long-term cannabidiol treatment in patients with Dravet syndrome : an open-label extension trial. *Epilepsia* 2019;60(2):294–302.

Devinsky O, Patel AD, Cross JH, et al. Effect of cannabidiol on drop seizures in the Lennox-Gastaut syndrome. *N Engl J Med* 2018;378(20):1888–97.

Devinsky O, Patel AD, Thiele EA, et al. Randomized, dose-ranging safety trial of cannabidiol in Dravet syndrome. *Neurology* 2018;90:e1204–11.

Devinsky O, Verducci C, Thiele EA, et al. Open-label use of highly purified CBD (Epidiolex®) in patients with CDKL5 deficiency disorder and Aicardi, Dup15q, and Doose syndromes. *Epilepsy Behav* 2018;86:131–7.

Dunwiddie TV. Endogenously released adenosine regulates excitability in the in vitro hippocampus. *Epilepsia* 1980;21(5):541–8.

El Marroun H, Bolhuis K, Franken IHA, et al. Preconception and prenatal cannabis use and the risk of behavioural and emotional problems in the offspring; a multi-informant prospective longitudinal study. *Int J Epidemiol* 2019;48(1):287–96.

ElSohly MA, Radwan MM, Gul W, Chandra S, Galal A. Phytochemistry of cannabis sativa l, progress in the chemistry of organic natural products. *Prog Chem Org Nat Prod* 2017;103:1–36.

EMCDDA. *Cannabis legislation in Europe. An overview.* 2018. http://www.emcdda.europa.eu/system/files/publications/4135/TD0217210ENN.pdf.

European Medicines Agency. *Epidyolex.* 2019. https://www.ema.europa.eu/en/medicines/human/EPAR/epidyolex.

FDA. FDA approves first drug comprised of an active ingredient derived from marijuana to treat rare, severe forms of epilepsy. 2018. https://www.fda.gov/newsevents/newsroom/pressannouncements/ucm611046.htm.

Filloux F. Cannabinoids for paediatric epilepsy? Up in smoke or real science? *Transl Pediatr* 2015;4:271–82.

Franco V, Perucca E. Pharmacological and therapeutic properties of cannabidiol for epilepsy. *Drugs* 2019;79(13):1435–54.

Fredholm BB, Chen JF, Cunha RA, Svenningsson P, Vaugeois JM. Adenosine and brain function. *Int Rev Neurobiol* 2005;63:191–270.

French National Agency for Medicines and Health Products Safety (ANSM). *Cannabis thérapeutique en France : l'ANSM publie les premières conclusions du CSST - Point d'Information.* 2018. https://www.ansm.sante.fr/S-informer/Points-d-information-Points-d-information/Cannabis-therapeutique-en-France-l-ANSM-publie-les-premieres-conclusions-du-CSST-Point-d-Information.

Friedman D, Devinsky O. Cannabinoids in the treatment of epilepsy. *N Engl J Med* 2016;374(1):94–5.

Gaston TE, Bebin EM, Cutter GR, et al. Interactions between cannabidiol and commonly used antiepileptic drugs. *Epilepsia* 2017;58:1586–92.

Gaston TE, Bebin EM, Cutter GR, Liu Y, Szarflarski JP. UAB CBD Program Interaction between cannabidiol and commonly used antiepileptic drugs. *Epilepsia* 2017;58(9):1586–92.

Geffrey AL, Pollack SF, Bruno PL, Thiele EA. Drug-drug interaction between clobazam and cannabidiol in children with refractory epilepsy. *Epilepsia* 2015;56(8):1246–51.

Ghovanloo MR, Shuart NG, Mezeyova J, Dean RA, Ruben PC, Goodchild SJ. Inhibitory effects of cannabidiol on voltage-dependent sodium currents. *J Biol Chem* 2018;293:16546–58.

GMC. *Consent: patients and doctors making decisions together.* 2008. https://www.gmc-uk.org/ethical-guidance/ethical-guidance-for-doctors/consent.

GMC. *Prescribing unlicensed medicines.* 2019. https://www.gmc-uk.org/ethical-guidance/ethical-guidance-for-doctors/prescribing-and-managing-medicines-and-devices/prescribing-unlicensed-medicines.

Gofshteyn JS, Wilfong A, Devinsky O, et al. Cannabidiol as a potential treatment for febrile infection-related epilepsy syndrome (FIRES) in the acute and chronic phase. *J Child Neurol* 2017;32(1):35–40.

Gordon AJ, Conley JW, Gordon JM. Medical consequences of marijuana use: a review of current literature. *Curr Psychiatry Rep* 2013;15(12):419.

Gray RA, Stott CG, Jones NJ, Di Marzo V, Whalley BJ. Anticonvulsive properties of cannabidiol (CBD) in a model of generalized seizure are transient receptor potential vanilloid 1 (TRPV1) dependent. Cannabis and Cannabinoid Research 2019. [Epub ahead of print].

Gray RA, Stott CG, Jones NJ, Wright S. The effect of a pharmaceutical formulation of cannabidiol on human cns-expressed voltage-gated sodium channels. *Neurology* 2017;88(16 Supplement):228. P1.

Gray RA, Whalley B. Working mechanisms of cannabinoids. *Epileptic Disord* 2020;22(Suppl. 1): S10–5.

Grewen K, Salzwedel AP, Gao W. Functional connectivity disruption in neonates with prenatal marijuana exposure. *Front Hum Neurosci* 2015;9:601.

Gross DW, Hamm J, Ashworth NL, Quigley D. Marijuana use and epilepsy: prevalence in patients of a tertiary care epilepsy center. *Neurology* 2004;62(11):2095–7.

Gunn JK, Rosales CB, Center KE, Nuñez AV, Gibson SJ, Ehiri JE. The effects of prenatal cannabis exposure on fetal development and pregnancy outcomes: a protocol. *BMJ Open* 2015;5(3): e007227.

Hamerle M, Ghaeni L, Kowski A, Weissinger F, Holtkamp M. Cannabis and other illicit drug use in epilepsy patients. *Eur J Neurol* 2014;21(1):167–70.

Hess EJ, Moody KA, Geffrey AL, et al. Cannabidiol as a new treatment for drug-resistant epilepsy in tuberous sclerosis complex. *Epilepsia* 2016;57(10):1617–24.

Hill AJ, Williams CM, Whalley BJ, Stephens GJ. Phytocannabinoids as novel therapeutic agents in CNS disorders. *Pharmacol Ther* 2012;133(1):79–97.

Holdcroft A, Maze M, Doré C, Tebbs S, Thompson S. A multicenter dose-escalation study of the analgesic and adverse effects of an oral cannabis extract (Cannador) for postoperative pain management. *Anesthesiology* 2006;104(5):1040–6.

Holdcroft A, Smith M, Jacklin A, et al. Pain relief with oral cannabinoids in familial Mediterranean fever. *Anaesthesia* 1997;52(5):483–6.

Hussain SA, Zhou R, Jacobson C, et al. Perceived efficacy of cannabidiol-enriched cannabis extracts for treatment of pediatric epilepsy: a potential role for infantile spasms and Lennox-Gastaut syndrome. *Epilepsy Behav* 2015;47:138–41.

Iannotti FA, Hill CL, Leo A, et al. Non-psychotropic plant cannabinoids, cannabidivarin (CBDV) and cannabidiol (CBD) activate and desensitize transient receptor potential vanilloid 1 (TRPV1) channels in vitro: potential for the treatment of neuronal hyperexcitability. *ACS Chem Neurosci* 2014;5:1131–41.

Ibeas Bih C, Chen T, Nunn AV, Bazelot M, Dallas M, Whalley BJ. Molecular targets of cannabidiol in neurological disorders. *Neurotherapeutics* 2015;12:699–730.

Johannessen Landmark C, Brandl U. Pharmacology and drug interactions of cannabinoids. *Epileptic Disord* 2020;22(Suppl. 1):S16–22.

Johannessen Landmark C, Johannessen SI, Tomson T. Dosing strategies for antiepileptic drugs: from a standard dose for all to individualised treatment by implementation of therapeutic drug monitoring. *Epileptic Disord* 2016;18:367–83.

Johannessen Landmark C, Johannessen SI, Tomson T. Host factors affecting antiepileptic drug delivery-Pharmacokinetic variability. *Adv Drug Deliv Rev* 2012;64:896–910.

Johannessen Landmark C, Johannessen SI. Drug safety aspects of antiepileptic drugs- focus on pharmacovigilance. *Pharmacoepidem Drug Saf* 2012;21:11–20.

Johannessen Landmark C, Patsalos PN. Drug interactions involving the new second and third generation antiepileptic drugs. *Exp Rev Neurother* 2010;10:119–40.

Johannessen SI, Johannessen Landmark C. Antiepileptic drug interactions-Basic principles and clinical implications. *Current Neuropharm* 2010;8:254–67.

Jones NA, Hill AJ, Smith I, et al. Cannabidiol displays antiepileptiform and antiseizure properties in vitro and in vivo. *J Pharmacol Exp Ther* 2010;332(2):569–77.

Kapur A, Zhao P, Sharir H, et al. Atypical responsiveness of the orphan receptor GPR55 to cannabinoid ligands. *J Biol Chem* 2009;284:29817–27.

Klein BD, et al. Evaluation of cannabidiol in animal seizure models by the Epilepsy Therapy Screening Program (ETSP). *Neurochem Res* 2017;42(7):1939–48.

Koppel BS, Brust JC, Fife T, et al. Systematic review: efficacy and safety of medical marijuana in selected neurologic disorders: report of the Guideline Development Subcommittee of the American Academy of Neurology. *Neurology* 2014;82:1556–63.

Lagae L. Long-term effects of cannabinoids on development/behavior. *Epileptic Disord* 2020;22(Suppl. 1):S33–37.

Lattanzi S, Brigo F, Cagnetti C, Trinka E, Silvestrini M. Efficacy and safety of adjunctive cannabidiol in patients with Lennox-Gastaut syndrome: a systematic review and meta-analysis. *CNS Drugs* 2018;32(10):905–16.

Lattanzi S, Brigo F, Trinka E, et al. Efficacy and safety of cannabidiol. a systematic review and meta-analysis. *Drugs* 2018;78:1791–804.

Laux LC, Bebin EM, Checketts D, et al. Long-term safety and efficacy of cannabidiol in children and adults with treatment resistant Lennox-Gastaut syndrome or Dravet syndrome: Expanded access program results. *Epilepsy Res* 2019;154:13–20.

Liou GI, Auchampach JA, Hillard CJ, et al. Mediation of cannabidiol anti-inflammation in the retina by equilibrative nucleoside transporter and A2A adenosine receptor. *Invest Ophthalmol Vis Sci* 2008;49:5526–31.

Lopez-Larson MP, Rogowska J, Yurgelun-Todd D. Aberrant orbitofrontal connectivity in marijuana smoking adolescents. *Dev Cogn Neurosci* 2015;16:54–62.

Lynch ME, Campbell F. Cannabinoids for treatment of chronic non-cancer pain; a systematic review of randomized trials. *Br J Clin Pharmacol* 2011;72(5):735–44.

Maa E, Figi P. The case for medical marijuana in epilepsy. *Epilepsia* 2014;55(6):783–6.

McCoy B, Wang L, Zak M, et al. A prospective open-label trial of a CBD/THC cannabis oil in Dravet syndrome. *Ann Clin Transl Neurol* 2018;5(9):1077–88.

Medicines and Healthcare products Regulatory Agency. *MHRA statement on products containing Cannabidiol (CBD)*. 2016. https://www.gov.uk/government/news/mhra-statement-on-products-containing-cannabidiol-cbd.

Meier MH, Caspi A, Ambler A, et al. Persistent cannabis users show neuropsychological decline from childhood to midlife. *Proc Natl Acad Sci USA* 2012;109(40):E2657–64.

Miech RA, Johnston LD, O'Malley PM, Bachman JG, Schulenberg JE, Patrick ME. *Monitoring the Future National Survey Results on Drug Use, 1975-2017: Volume I, Secondary School Students*. Ann Arbor: Institute for Social Research, The University of Michigan, 2018: 566.

Mijangos-Moreno S, Poot-Aké A, Arankowsky-Sandoval G, Murillo-Rodríguez E. Intrahypothalamic injection of cannabidiol increases the extracellular levels of adenosine in nucleus accumbens in rats. *Neurosci Res* 2014;84:60–3.

Millar SA, Stone NL, Yates AS, O'Sullivan SE. A systematic review on the pharmacokinetics of cannabidiol in humans. *Front Pharmacol* 2018;9:1–13.

Miller I, Perry S, Saneto R, et al. Cannabidiol (CBD; 10 and 20 mg/kg/day) significantly reduces convulsive seizure frequency in children and adolescents with Dravet syndrome (DS): Results of a dose-ranging, multicenter, randomized, double-blind, placebo-controlled trial (GWPCARE2). *Neurology* 2019;93(5):e532.

Mori F, Ribolsi M, Kusayanagi H, et al. TRPV1 channels regulate cortical excitability in humans. *J Neurosci* 2012;32(3):873–9.

Morrison G, Crockett J, Blakey G, Sommerville K. A Phase 1, Open-Label, Pharmacokinetic Trial to Investigate Possible Drug-Drug Interactions Between Clobazam, Stiripentol, or Valproate and Cannabidiol in Healthy Subjects. *Clin Pharmacol Drug Dev* 2019;8(8):1009–31.

Müller-Vahl KR. Treatment of Tourette syndrome with cannabinoids. *Behav Neurol* 2013;27(1):119–24.

Nabbout R, Thiele E. The role of cannabinoids in epilepsy treatment: a critical review of efficacy results from clinical trials. *Epileptic Disord* 2020;22(Suppl. 1):S23–8.

New Zealand Government Ministry of Health. *Search results for medicinal cannabis.* 2017. https://www.health.govt.nz/search/results/medicinal_cannabis.

NICE. *Cannabis-based medicinal products.* 2019. https://www.nice.org.uk/guidance/ng144.

Nichol K, Stott C, Jones N, Gray R, Bazelot M, Whalley BJ. *The proposed multimodal mechanism of action of cannabidiol (cbd) in epilepsy: modulation of intracellular calcium and adenosine-mediated signaling.* Abst. 2.462. American Epilepsy Society, 2018.

Noyes R Jr, Brunk SF, Baram DA, Canter A. Analgesic effect of delta-9-tetrahydrocannabinol. *J Clin Pharmacol* 1975;15(2–3):139–43.

Pamplona FA, da Silva LR, Coan AC. Potential clinical benefits of CBD-rich cannabis extracts over purified CBD in treatment-resistant epilepsy: observational data meta-analysis. *Front Neurol* 2018;12(9):759.

Patel RR, Barbosa C, Brustovetsky T, Brustovetsky N, Cummins TR. Aberrant epilepsy-associated mutant Nav1.6 sodium channel activity can be targeted with cannabidiol. *Brain* 2016;139:2164–81.

Patsalos PN, Berry DJ, Bourgeois BF, et al. Antiepileptic drugs-best practice guidelines for therapeutic drug monitoring: a position paper by the subcommission on therapeutic drug monitoring, ILAE Commission on Therapeutic Strategies. *Epilepsia* 2008;49:1239–76.

Patsalos PN, Spencer EP, Berry DJ. Therapeutic drug monitoring of antiepileptic drugs in epilepsy: a 2018 update. *Ther Drug Monit* 2018;40:526–48.

Patsalos PN, Zugman M, Lake C, James A, Ratnaraj N, Sander JW. Serum protein binding of 25 antiepileptic drugs in a routine clinical setting: A comparison of free non-protein-bound concentrations. *Epilepsia* 2017;58(7):1234–43.

Patsalos PN. Drug interactions with the newer antiepileptic drugs (AEDs)-Part 1: pharmacokinetic and pharmacodynamic interactions between AEDs. *Clin Pharmacokinet* 2013;52:927–66.

Patsalos PN. Drug interactions with the newer antiepileptic drugs (AEDs)-Part 2: pharmacokinetic and pharmacodynamic interactions between AEDs and drugs used to treat non-epilepsy disorders. *Clin Pharmacokinet* 2013;52(12):1045–61.

Patsalos PN. Drug interactions with the newer antiepileptic drugs (AEDs)-Part 1: pharmacokinetic and pharmacodynamic interactions between AEDs. *Clin Pharmacokinet* 2013;52:927–66.

Pavlovic R, Nenna G, Calvi L. Quality traits of "cannabidiol oils": cannabinoids content, terpene fingerprint and oxidation stability of European commercially available preparations. *Molecules* 2018;20(2):5.

Pegoraro CN, Nutter D, Thevenon M, Ramirez CL. Chemical profiles of cannabis sativa medicinal oil using different extraction and concentration methods. *Nat Prod Res* 2019;12:1–4.

Perucca E. Cannabinoids in the treatment of epilepsy: hard evidence at last? *J Epilepsy Res* 2017;7(2):61–76.

Pisanti S, Malfitano AM, Ciaglia E, et al. Cannabidiol: state of the art and new challenges for therapeutic applications. *Pharmacol Ther* 2017;175:133–50.

Porcari GS, Fu C, Doll ED, Carter EG, Carson RP. Efficacy of artisanal preparations of cannabidiol for the treatment of epilepsy: practical experiences in a tertiary medical center. *Epilepsy Behav* 2018;80:240–6.

Porter BE, Jacobson C. Report of a parent survey of cannabidiol-enriched cannabis use in pediatric treatment-resistant epilepsy. *Epilepsy Behav* 2013;29(3):574–7.

Press CA, Knupp KG, Chapman KE. Parental reporting of response to oral cannabis extracts for treatment of refractory epilepsy. *Epilepsy Behav* 2015;45:49–52.

Ribeiro A, Ferraz-de-Paula V, Pinheiro ML, et al. Cannabidiol, a non-psychotropic plant-derived cannabinoid, decreases inflammation in a murine model of acute lung injury : role for the adenosine A(2A) receptor. *Eur J Pharmacol* 2012;678(1–3):78–85.

Robbins MS, Tarshish S, Solomon S, Grosberg BM. Cluster attacks responsive to recreational cannabis and dronabinol. *Headache* 2009;49(6):914–6.

Roberts JC, Davis JB, Benham CD. [3H]Resiniferatoxin autoradiography in the CNS of wild-type and TRPV1 null mice defines TRPV1 (VR-1) protein distribution. *Brain Res* 2004;995:176–83.

Rong C, Lee Y, Carmona NE, et al. Cannabidiol in medical marijuana: research vistas and potential opportunities. *Pharmacol Res* 2017;121:213–8.

Rosenberg E, Bazelot M, Chamberland S, et al. *Cannabidiol (CBD) exerts anti-epileptic actions by targeting the LPI-GPR55 signaling system potentiated by seizures*. Abstr. 3. 052. American Epilepsy Society 2018.

Rosenberg EC, Louik J, Conway E, Devinsky O, Friedman D. Quality of Life in Childhood Epilepsy in pediatric patients enrolled in a prospective, open-label clinical study with cannabidiol. *Epilepsia* 2017;58(8):e96–100.

Rosenberg EC, Patra PH, Whalley BJ. Therapeutic effects of cannabinoids in animal models of seizures, epilepsy, epileptogenesis, and epilepsy-related neuroprotection. *Epilepsy Behav* 2017;70 (Pt B):319–27.

Rubino T, Parolaro D. The impact of exposure to cannabinoids in adolescence : insights from animal models. *Biol Psychiatry* 2016;79(7):578–85.

Russo EB. Cannabinoids in the management of difficult to treat pain. *Ther Clin Risk Manag* 2008;4(1):245–59.

Russo EB, Taming THC. Potential cannabis synergy and phytocannabinoid-terpenoid entourage effects. *Br J Pharmacol* 2011;163:1344–64.

Ryberg E, Larsson N, Sjögren S, et al. The orphan receptor GPR55 is a novel cannabinoid receptor. *Br J Pharmacol* 2007;152(7):1092–101.

Sabaz M, Lawson JA, Cairns DR, et al. Validation of the quality of life in childhood epilepsy questionnaire in American epilepsy patients. *Epilepsy Behav* 2003;4(6):680–91.

Santiago M, Sachdev S, Arnold JC, McGregor IS, Connor M. Absence of Entourage: Terpenoids Commonly Found in Cannabis sativa Do Not Modulate the Functional Activity of Δ9-THC at Human CB1 and CB2 Receptors. *Cannabis Cannabinoid Res* 2019;4(3):165–76.

Sawzdargo M, Nguyen T, Lee DK, et al. Identification and cloning of three novel human G protein-coupled receptor genes GPR52, PsiGPR53 and GPR55: GPR55 is extensively expressed in human brain. *Brain Res Mol Brain Res* 1999;64:193–8.

Schonhofen P, Bristot IJ, Crippa JA. Cannabinoid-based therapies and brain development: potential harmful effect of early modulation of the endocannabinoid system. *CNS Drugs* 2018;32(8):697–712.

Sebastião AM, Macedo MP, Ribeiro JA. Tonic activation of A(2A) adenosine receptors unmasks, and of A(1) receptors prevents, a facilitatory action of calcitonin gene-related peptide in the rat hippocampus. *Br J Pharmacol* 2000;129(2):374–80.

Sebastiao AM, Ribeiro JA. Adenosine receptors and the central nervous system. *Handb Exp Pharmacol* 2009;193:471–534.

Sharir H, Abood ME. Pharmacological characterization of GPR55, a putative cannabinoid receptor. *Pharmacol Ther* 2010;126:301–13.

Skrabek RQ, Galimova L, Ethans K, Perry D. Nabilone for the treatment of pain in fibromyalgia. *J Pain* 2008;9(2):164–73.

Smith LA, Azariah F, Lavender VT, Stoner NS, Bettiol S. Cannabinoids for nausea and vomiting in adults with cancer receiving chemotherapy. *Cochrane Database Syst Rev* 2015;12(11). CD009464.

Sparrow SS, Cicchetti DV. Diagnostic uses of the Vineland Adaptive Behavior Scales. *J Pediatr Psychol* 1985;10(2):215–25.

Specchio N, Pietrafusa N, Cross HJ. Source of cannabinoids: what is available, what is used, and where does it come from? *Epileptic Disord* 2020;22(Suppl. 1):S1–9.

Stout SM, Cimino NM. Exogenous cannabinoids as substrates, inhibitors, and inducers of human drug metabolizing enzymes: a systematic review. *Drug Metab Rev* 2014;46(1):86–95.

Sun FJ, Guo W, Zheng DH, et al. Increased expression of TRPV1 in the cortex and hippocampus from patients with mesial temporal lobe epilepsy. *J Mol Neurosci* 2013;49(1):182–93.

Swiss Agency for Therapeutic Products. *Search results for CBD*. 2017. https://www.swissmedic.ch/swissmedic/en/home/suche.html#CBD.

Szaflarski JP, Bebin EM, Comi AM, et al. Long-term safety and treatment effects of cannabidiol in children and adults with treatment-resistant epilepsies: expanded access program results. *Epilepsia* 2018;59(8):1540–8.

Taylor L, Gidal B, Blakey G, Tayo B, Morrison G. A Phase I, randomized, double-blind, placebo-controlled, single ascending dose, multiple dose, and food effect trial of the safety, tolerability and pharmacokinetics of highly purified cannabidiol in healthy subjects. *CNS Drugs* 2018;32:1053–67.

Thiele E, Bebin M, Hari Bhathal H, et al. Cannabidiol (CBD) Treatment in Patients with Seizures Associated with Tuberous Sclerosis Complex: A Randomized, Double-blind, Placebo-Controlled Phase 3 Trial (GWPCARE6). AES meeting, Baltimore 2019.

Thiele E, Marsh E, Mazurkiewicz-Beldzinska M. Cannabidiol in patients with Lennox-Gastaut syndrome: interim analysis of an open-label extension study. *Epilepsia* 2019;60(3):419–28.

Thiele EA, Marsh ED, French JA, et al. Cannabidiol in patients with seizures associated with Lennox-Gastaut syndrome (GWPCARE4): a randomised, double-blind, placebo-controlled phase 3 trial. *Lancet* 2018;391(10125):1085–96.

Tomida I, Azuara-Blanco A, House H, et al. Effect of sublingual application of cannabinoids on intraocular pressure: a pilot study. *J Glaucoma* 2006;15(5):349–53.

Tortoriello G, Morris CV, Alpar A, et al. Miswiring the brain: delta9-tetra-hydrocannabinol disrupts cortical development by inducing an SCG10/stathmin-2 degradation pathway. *EMBO J* 2014;33(7):668–85.

Tóth A, Boczan J, Kedei N, et al. Expression and distribution of vanilloid receptor 1 (TRPV1) in the adult rat brain. *Brain Res Mol Brain Res* 2005;135:162–8.

Trembly B, Sherman, M. *Double-blind clinical study of cannabidiol as a secondary anticonvulsant*. Paper presented at Marijuana '90 Int. Conf. on Cannabis and Cannabinoids, Kolympari (Crete), 1990; July 8-11.

Tzadok M, Uliel-Siboni S, Linder I. CBD-enriched medical cannabis for intractable pediatric epilepsy: the current Israeli experience. *Seizure* 2016;35:41–4.

Ujvary I, Hanus L. Human metabolites of cannabidiol: a review on their formation, biological activity, and relevance in therapy. *Cannabis Cannabinoid Res* 2016;1:90–101.

Vandrey R, Raber JC, Raber ME, Douglass B, Miller C, Bonn-Miller MO. Cannabinoid dose and label accuracy in edible medical cannabis products. *JAMA* 2015;313(24):2491–3.

Weltha L, Reemmer J, Boison D. The role of adenosine in epilepsy. *Brain Res Bull* 2019;151:46–54.

Whiting PF, Wolff RF, Deshpande S, et al. Cannabinoids for medical use: a systematic review and meta-analysis. *JAMA* 2015;313(24):2456–73.

Xing J, Li J. TRPV1 receptor mediates glutamatergic synaptic input to dorsolateral periaqueductal gray (dl-PAG) neurons. *J Neurophysiol* 2007;97:503–11.

Yamamoto Y, Takahashi Y, Imai K, et al. Influence of CYP2C19 polymorphism and concomitant antiepileptic drugs on serum clobazam and N-desmethylclobazam concentrations in patients with epilepsy. *Ther Drug Monit* 2013;35(3):305–12.

Zaami S, Di Luca A, Di Luca NM, Montanari Vergallo G. Medical use of cannabis: Italian and European legislation. *Eur Rev Med Pharmacol Sci* 2018;22:1161–7.